INTERROGATING PREGNANCY LOSS

Funded by the Government of Canada
Financé par la gouvernement du Canada | Canadä

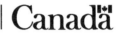

Demeter Press
140 Holland Street West
P. O. Box 13022
Bradford, ON L3Z 2Y5
Tel: (905) 775-9089
Email: info@demeterpress.org
Website: www.demeterpress.org

Demeter Press logo based on the sculpture "Demeter" by Maria-Luise Bodirsky
www.keramik-atelier.bodirsky.de

Printed and Bound in Canada

Front cover artwork: Mindy Stricke "Crabapples," from the project *Grief Landscapes*, 2016, Digital photograph. www.mindystricke.com.

Library and Archives Canada Cataloguing in Publication

        Interrogating pregnancy loss : feminist writings on abortion, miscarriage and stillbirth / edited by Emily R.M. Lind and Angie Deveau.

Includes bibliographical references.
ISBN 978-1-77258-023-5 (softcover)

        1. Feminism. 2. Pregnancy. 3. Abortion. 4. Miscarriage. 5. Stillbirth. 6. Reproductive rights. I. Lind, Emily R. M., 1981-, editor II. Deveau, Angie, 1979-, editor

HQ1155.I58 2017   305.42   C2017-906163-1

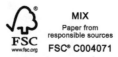

MIX
Paper from
responsible sources
FSC® C004071

INTERROGATING PREGNANCY LOSS

Feminist Writings on Abortion, Miscarriage, and Stillbirth

EDITED BY

Emily R. M. Lind and Angie Deveau

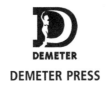

DEMETER

DEMETER PRESS

MINDY STRICKE, ARTIST STATEMENT

> *Grief is like a long valley, a winding valley where any bend may reveal a totally new landscape.*
>
> —C.S. Lewis, *A Grief Observed*

The cover image, "Crabapples," is a photograph from Grief Landscapes, by artist Mindy Stricke. Grief Landscapes is collaborative art project that combines real people's personal stories and evocative macro photographs to document the wide varieties of ways people respond to and learn to live with loss. Grief is often described as a journey, but it's an intensely individual and often isolating one: rarely do people speak openly about the range of ways of grieving, and there are many misconceptions about the grief process.

Mindy Stricke developed the project in a public online process after her close friend lost her young son, as a way to help her friend feel less alone in her grief. Inspired by the C.S. Lewis quote above, she set out to visually record people's unique grief "landscapes" by inviting the public to submit their experiences with bereavement, and then photographing an object in close-up related to each story. Each object was transformed into an abstract landscape, capturing the emotional intensity of each piece through the image.

Crabapples is one of the forty stories and images in the body of work, made in response to Nadia Obrigewitsch's experience of losing her daughter Aida at birth. To read Nadia's full story, go to http://www.mindystricke.com.

I dedicate this collection to Christopher Ruth Gordon Lind,
born still on 15 April 2017.
You remain one of my most precious stories.
—Emma

To my one and only Sam:
My love for you is unfathomable. While you are still only six,
I hope that one day you'll be able to read these stories and
deeply appreciate the love, heartache, and loss
that we have experienced. And please keep that wonderful
sense of humour of yours—you can always make me laugh,
even in my saddest moments.
—Angie

Table of Contents

Acknowledgements

Andrea O'Reilly's inspired enthusiasm for this project gave it shape in the early stages, and we would like to thank her for her encouragement, and her belief in us as editors. The Motherhood Initiative for Research and Community Involvement (MIRCI) has facilitated new directions in our thinking over the years, and without the opportunities to think, struggle, and publish alongside other MIRCI scholars, we would not have been able to imagine this collection as a possibility. Special thanks to May Friedman for her insights on pregnancy loss as well as her gracious mentorship in bringing a project to completion with Demeter Press.

We also have deep gratitude for the friends, colleagues, and family who offered their never-ending support over the past few years—whether it was to lend an ear as we fleshed out ideas and frustrations with finding the words, or offered their advice.

Emma: I would like to thank Matthew J. Trafford, Adrienne Gruber, Brecken Hancock, Samantha Cutrara, Andrea Flowers, Liz Nelson, Karin Galldin, May Friedman, Claire Carter, Allyson Marsolais, Kim de Bellefeuille-Percy, and Stefanie Hurst who rallied generous levels of wisdom and offered them up, enabling me to interrogate pregnancy loss long enough to find my way home. Deep thanks to my mother and stepfather, Heather Musgrove and Rene Roy, for feeding and housing me as this book was completed. And for sharing my loss as your own. The day this book was sent for peer review, I gave birth to my stillborn son, Christopher. I would like to acknowledge Marissa Charbonneau, Rosemarie Parisien, Chantal Bourbonnais, and Victoria Kellett for supporting me through labour and delivery. It is because of you that Christopher's birth is not just a tragic story. His birth is also a powerful, beautiful, and important story, and the roles you played (so well!) gave me the strength to continue with this project and push it out.

Angie: I would like to thank my partner, Bob, and my son, Sam, for their patience as I worked on this project. I would also like to thank Elizabeth Saunders, Jessica Webster, and Kerri Goodwin for being there for me in my greatest time of need. Lastly, I want to thank Dr. Deborah Harrison for always believing in my abilities—both as an undergraduate student and beyond.

Lastly, we would like to thank the contributors for their patience in putting this collection together, and their bravery in sharing their stories and research. Without their input, there would be no book.

Introduction

Toward a Feminist Epistemology of Loss

EMILY R. M. LIND

This project was born out of heartbreak—the heartbreak of our experiences of pregnancy loss and those of our friends and colleagues, all living with the pain of having lost what was promising (or threatening) to become. As feminist scholars, we found it nearly impossible to experience pregnancy loss—with its attendant gendered assumptions, mythologies, and identity conflicts—without also grappling with an understanding of how our experience of loss was embedded in the nexus of social power relations we have committed our lives to studying. The book in your hands is the product of that grappling. It interrogates pregnancy loss from a feminist perspective and asks most fundamentally: what can we know from what we've lost?

This collection imagines loss as an epistemological phenomenon—one that produces knowledge about the world and the bodies that inhabit it. Pregnancy loss can be too easily characterized by absence, lack, and biomedical exceptionalism. Here, we work to re-story such tropes toward an understanding of loss as productive, insightful, and, tragically, common. When we refer to loss, we speak beyond the parameters of loss as grief or as lack. As Kate Parsons asserts:

> Loss, whether intentional or unintentional, need not be restricted to those experiences about which a woman is upset or grief stricken. Although the term *loss* typically accompanies emotions of sadness or regret...it does not always do so. One of the most celebrated forms of *loss* in

our culture is weight loss... likewise, the loss of the placental organ is an event that inspires reverence and ritual. (14-15, emphasis in original)

Pregnancy *loss*, of course, stands in stark contrast to the expected outcome of reproduction: *gain*. By interrogating loss, this collection argues that the lessons learned from loss have the capacity to serve collective understandings of both loss and gain and of both the expected and unexpected rhythms of social and reproductive life. As Kirsten Hudson explores in her study of abortion, "the pregnant body and the maternal body are seen as interchangeable terms" (41). Just as scholars of maternal subjectivity have pushed for a broader definition of motherhood—one that accounts for adoptive motherhood, an enlarged scope of what constitutes maternal labour, and trans-inclusive parenting models—so too must feminist scholars disentangle the pregnancy-maternity association in an effort to theorize pregnancy as ontologically divorced from the inevitability of a live birth. As Hudson explains:

By conflating pregnant and maternal embodiment, women (and men) become locked into a narrative script that lacks room for thinking about the unique bodily perspective that emerges from experiences that deviate from such a singular linear trajectory. What talk there is of failed births, "bad" outcomes and absent lives seems cursory, obligatory, brief. (46)

This collection centres pregnancy loss as an embodied and social phenomenon within a framework that understands pregnancy as a process with no guaranteed outcomes. *Interrogating Pregnancy Loss* considers pregnancy as an epistemic source, one that has the capacity to reveal the limits of our collective assumptions about temporality, expectation, narrative, and social legitimacy.

GRIEF AND FEMINIST EPISTEMOLOGY

Rachel A.J. Hurst's work on the relationship between grief and feminist pedagogy informs this collection's focus on pregnancy loss as instructive. Reflecting on the presence of grief in a classroom, Hurst has argued that "the world is a wounded and hurting world shrouded in grief ... and the classroom can never be a space that is protected from loss" (Hurst 34). Similarly, this collection explores pregnancy as a state of being embedded in the dynamics of grief and loss that the following pages explore. These dynamics can constitute Alice Pitt and Deborah Britzman's definition of "difficult knowledge," which reflects both the study of trauma and the experience of it (qtd. in Hurst 40). The concept of "difficult knowledge" serves as a compelling reminder of how the affective stakes in our own personal histories are embedded in the epistemic tasks of understanding the social role of emotional pain. Hurst highlights Britzman's discussion of the distinction between learning about something and learning from it: "When we learn *about* something, we obtain a collection of facts...learning *from* belongs to the terrain of insight and of thinking of how the learner is interpolated and affected by knowledge" (Hurst 40, emphasis in original). We have assembled this collection knowing that pregnancy loss is often *learned about.* In an effort to *learn from* it, this collection considers how pregnancy loss requires a more Althusserian relationship to loss: rather being interpolated by it, we seek to understand the particularly subjective implications of loss. In other words, how are reproductive subjects inter*pellated* by it?

Fundamentally, this collection embraces a feminist approach to the study of pregnancy loss that "appreciates the sociopolitical context in which the loss is embedded" (Cosgrove 116). In the current sociopolitical context, reproductive rights are currently under threat of being constrained or curtailed in many North American jurisdictions where access to abortion on demand is legal. This collection draws together stories and studies that would have been conventionally presented in siloed formats. Abortion, miscarriage, and stillbirth are rarely studied together as phenomena linked by common themes. Given that abortion, miscarriage, and stillbirth could conceivably happen to the same person over the course of a reproductive lifetime, that patients carrying nonviable pregnancies are sometimes offered a dilation and curettage (D&C) to expedite the process, and that clinical categories of pregnancy loss (for instance, "spontaneous" versus "therapeutic" abortions) share very similar names—the research convention of studying these events as distinctive rather than interrelated reveals an epistemic limitation of the field. Certainly, this categorical distinction in research is due in part to the need for specific knowledge and expertise regarding each form of pregnancy loss. However, isolating the study of abortion from studies of miscarriage and stillbirth is also informed by what Linda Layne has called the "studied silence" ("Breaking the Silence" 294) that feminist scholars maintain regarding abortion as a form of loss, for fear of reproducing the antichoice discourse of fetal personhood. A vast literature contends with the moral and legal considerations regarding the "personhood debates" in the study of abortion rights (McLeod; Sherwin; Steinbock; Thompson; Warren). We are neither reopening nor contributing to these debates. This collection is organized around the feminist imperative to support and defend reproductive choice, and seeks to expand the ways those choices are understood as significant.

LITERATURE REVIEW

By compiling essays exploring abortion, miscarriage, and stillbirth in the same collection, we build upon the approach taken by Sarah Earle et al. in the only other book with a similar scope, *Understanding Reproductive Loss*. Earle et al. posit that by including studies of abortion alongside studies of other forms of reproductive loss, they reject the hierarchy of mourning that "categorises experiences of loss in a way that some might be seen as more 'serious' or 'traumatic' than others" (*Understanding* 2). We similarly reject the hierarchy of mourning that assigns more or less significance to forms of pregnancy loss depending on the stage of fetal development. Such an approach risks creating not only a hierarchy of mourning but a philosophical hierarchy between fetus and pregnant subject, which discerns the level of consequence based on fetal maturity alone. Although Earle et al.'s volume explores reproductive loss,[1] this collection takes on a more limited scope and focuses specifically on the loss of pregnancy, in an effort to resituate the gestating subject at the centre of our feminist examination of pregnancy loss.

Existing studies of pregnancy loss inevitably grapple with themes of thwarted expectations and unhappy endings—a consequence of the role pregnancy plays as a symbol of hope and futurity. Pregnancy loss is often studied from the perspective of grief and bereavement because studies of human reproduction are oriented toward the notion of reproductive success (Earle et al., "Conceptualizing Reproductive Loss"). Indeed, the cultural assumption that pregnancy leads to an inevitable live birth has been proven to aggravate the pain of pregnancy loss (Layne, *Motherhood Lost*). Because pregnancy has been conceptualized as a future-oriented process resulting in a baby, when pregnancy ends otherwise, it is labelled a "failure" (Letherby 165). Since gendered ideologies promote motherhood as true or idealized womanhood, many experience "failed" pregnancies as evidence of failing to conform to gendered expectations (Cacciatore and Bushfield; Davidson and Letherby; Davidson and Stahls; Earle et al., *Understanding*; Layne, *Motherhood*; Letherby). Furthermore, pregnancy loss can be experienced as a life-course disruption (Earle et al. "Social Dimensions"; Earle and Letherby). Therefore, the loss of parental subjectivity is a significant theme emerging from studies of pregnancy loss. In particular, stillbirth can create "an abrupt cut off in the identity construction process" especially when the "denial of the baby's existence was expressed" (Lovell 760). These themes are echoed in the literature about miscarriage (Letherby; Gerber-Epstein et al.). One strategy for recovering parental identity and claiming discursive space for the loss is to refer to the lost pregnancy as a lost "baby" (Parsons). This creates an epistemological tension within feminist studies, as reproductive choice is implicitly called into question when fetal personhood is asserted. As Linda Layne has argued, "the issue of pregnancy loss...poses a challenge for feminist scholars and activists ... to take an active part in constructing a more liberatory discourse of pregnancy loss" ("Breaking the Silence" 310).

FEMINIST MODELS FOR INTERROGATING PREGNANCY LOSS

What would a more "liberatory discourse" look like, then, for studying pregnancy loss? Is it possible to consider the autonomy of the pregnant subject while also making room, conceptually, for the idea of a lost "baby" in the shadow of grief? Is there a framework flexible enough to contend with the difficult truth that feelings of devastation and relief may be experienced in the context of loss? Or that some pregnancy endings involve lost "babies" and others the loss of reproductive tissue? And where are our bodies in all of this? Do we lose (or gain?) parts of ourselves as the potential body of another leaves our body, or the bodies of our friends, family members, surrogates, and partners?

Layne argues that feminists should adopt an "anthropologically informed view of personhood, that is, that personhood is culturally constructed ... one can see that the process of constructing personhood may be undertaken with some embryos and not others" ("Breaking the Silence" 305). Using this model, parents who plan for intended children—who name them and prepare space in their home to house them—develop what William Ruddick calls a "proleptic relationship ... treating the future state of affairs as if it already existed" (qtd. in Lindemann 84). Understanding personhood as culturally constructed opens up ontological room to privilege the social process by which personhood is constructed rather than assigning personhood based on stages of biological development alone. An anthropologically informed notion of personhood invites pregnancy itself to be considered outside of a strictly physical framework, enabling considerations into how parental subjectivity is similarly culturally constructed. Just as fetal personhood gets slowly constructed over the course of pregnancy through the labour of anticipation and preparation, so too could parental subjectivity emerge as a process built socially and culturally (a productive conceptual tool, especially when considering the construction of parental identity for nonbiological parents). The process of interrogating pregnancy loss inevitably includes an examination of how parental identity has been lost or called into question, engaging with themes that hold implications for studies of infertility and non-normative family structures.

Kate Parsons' notion of a "relational" model of pregnancy loss provides a complementary conceptual model for interrogating loss from a feminist perspective. Her description of the model is worth quoting at length:

On a relational model of pregnancy (and of pregnancy loss) as I conceive it, a woman and her fetus are physically connected beings, but there are contingent and severable aspects of this connection. One can conceptualize, name, and define a [person] and their embryo/fetus as physically connected to each other, while still recognizing the variability in [people's] emotional and intellectual connections to their fetuses. We can conceptualize a woman and her embryo/fetus as interrelated on a physical level, while still recognizing the severability of that relationship, attaching as little or as much emotional significance to the relationship as each woman deems fit.... Such a model, I believe, appreciates the dependence of the embryo/fetus on the woman, and the ways in which the woman and the embryo/fetus are growing and developing together. (12)

Applying Parsons's model enables pregnant subjects the autonomy to name and determine the significance of their relationship to the fetus. This framework supports abortion as a morally valid choice and enables pregnant people to know the fetus inside of them as a "baby." Parsons cites feminist theorists such as Donna Haraway, Elizabeth Grosz, Helene Cixous, and Luce Irigaray for having theorized pregnancy as an interrelational state of being, demonstrating how the pregnant body is not fixed but rather "shifting, permeable, expandable [and] unresolvable" (Parsons 13). Considering how to apply a relational model of pregnancy loss, Parsons offers the following:

On a relational reconceptualization, my losses could be understood more holistically, not merely as the death of developing beings, but also as the loss of my hopes and expectations, as well as fluids and tissue, that I built up in the pregnancy. My miscarriages on this model become "pregnancy losses" not merely embryonic/fetal losses, with a much fuller conception of pregnancy than that of containing, housing or carrying an embryo/fetus. (14)

This collection engages with the models proposed by Layne and

Parsons; as editors, we understand pregnancy loss as a subject that is "epistemologically opaque" (Lindemann 88) because no two pregnancy losses are socially, morally, or physically equivalent. In the words of feminist ethicist Susan Sherwin, "Fetuses develop in specific pregnancies which occur in the lives of particular women … their very existence is relational, developing as they do within particular … bodies, and their principal relationship is to the women who carry them" (243). In order to explore the particularities of any given loss and to understand what makes the loss of a specific pregnancy significant, scholars must center the voices of pregnant people. This approach is echoed by the legacy and sustained tradition of feminists theorizing the legitimacy of reproductive choice, as much as it is corroborated by findings within pregnancy loss literature that show bereaved parents "want authority over their own grief" (Davidson and Stahls 22).

THIS COLLECTION

This collection contains personal stories as well as studies of stories told about pregnancy loss. Stories are tools that help us understand our physical selves, or what Hilde Lindemann has called "narrative tissue," which allows us to "navigate the social world" (80). By interrogating the stories told about pregnancy loss, many of the authors in this collection engage in what Gayle Letherby and Deborah Davidson call "theorized subjectivity" (345). Theorized subjectivity "requires the constant, critical interrogation of our personhood—both intellectual and personal—within the production of knowledge, which starts by recognizing the value … of the subjective" (345).

Section One, "Breaking the Silence," features three chapters articulating the extent to which pregnancy loss is experienced as internalized feelings of shame and personal failure. As Layne has argued, "Both [biomedical and holistic approaches to pregnancy loss] are based on, and propagate, the belief that reproduction is something that can and should be controlled" ("Unhappy Endings" 1885). Furthermore, she argues that "the ethic of individual control is embedded in a culture of meritocracy" ("Unhappy Endings" 1888). Consequently, "the discursive space for pregnancy loss ... that contradict our cherished narratives of progress remains hidden, taking place behind closed doors" ("Unhappy Endings" 1889). The chapters in this section speak back to the cultural silences and the silencing myths of personal responsibility, biological inadequacy, and legitimized grief. Masha Sukovic and Margie Serrato's "Communicating Miscarriage: Coping with Loss, Uncertainty, and Self-Imposed Stigma" share their stories of miscarriage as "sense-making devices ... as tools to repair and heal our identities ... and as vehicles to communicate our stories to other women and those who care for them." They tell stories that differ from each other, but both share the common theme that prior to miscarriage, they found themselves "trapped in the delusion of effortless perfection, because we believed that we were in control over the creation of the perfect reproductive environment for our babies to grow in." To reclaim their sense of personal agency, the authors conclude that miscarriage is "inherently uncontrollable." Having clarified that miscarriage can function as a "stigmatizing illness," they insist on communicating and co-creating personal narratives of loss in order to enter the "new spaces of self-realization and self-acceptance." Similarly, in "Timeline of a Maternal Breakdown: A Feminist Mother's Blog Post About Her Abortion Experience," Angie Deveau chronicles her experience of abortion to counter the culture of silence surrounding the decision to terminate a pregnancy. She writes: "And this is why I have decided to tell my story. I want to help other women who may be going through a similar experience. I want them to know that it is okay to grieve or not to grieve. It is okay to be disappointed in yourself or be depressed, but it's also okay to think that it was merely a mistake and you can move on with your life." Finally, Nancy Gerber's "Grief, and Shame, and Miscarriage" asserts that silence exacerbates the shame of miscarriage, which she hopes will diminish as intergenerational feminist dialogues allow younger generations to feel less isolated in their grief. By telling the story of her miscarriage, Gerber works to further an understanding of grief as an "acceptable and legitimate" response to miscarriage.

Section Two, "Pregnancy as Relational," contains three chapters exploring the relational dynamics of pregnancy and pregnancy loss. Just as Parsons has argued that a relational model for understanding pregnancy asserts the pregnant subject and the fetus are growing together, the next three chapters consider what knowledge is made possible through such growth. Mary Thompson's "Believing Is Seeing Is Believing: Elective Abortion and Visual Closure" examines the practice in some abortion clinics of allowing patients to view their postabortion tissue. For some, this can be a helpful tool to "counter the dominant (antiabortion) visual rhetoric of fetal representation." Thompson argues that the practice of allowing abortion patients to view their own fetal tissue enables them to explore the subjugated knowledge of their own fetus and make sense of its loss. Her essay inserts maternal subjectivity into the visual representation of fetuses and analyzes pregnancy and abortion as relational states. Whereas Thompson's chapter focuses on the material tangibility of pregnancy loss, Maya Bhave argues that in the context of stillbirth, maternal and fetal subjectivity exist intangibly. In her chapter "The Ambiguous Space of Motherhood: The Experience of Stillbirth," Bhave writes, "We do not make ourselves mothers; rather, our children construct us.... Motherhood cannot be conceptualized as just having a child on the floor eating cheerios ... motherhood comes in many forms." For Bhave, the experience of stillbirth offers an opportunity to consider motherhood in a redefined scope, and understand stillborn children as "about possibility and belief, not about tangibility and physical space." In "Full Circle: Exploring the Maternal Ambivalence of a Motherless Daughter," Natalie Morning similarly articulates the ambiguous space she finds herself in as a "childless motherless daughter." She writes the following: "At times, when attempting to conceptualize motherhood, I feel as if I am not entitled to an opinion.... Maternal ambivalence, abortion, and maternal bereavement are not only associated with absence but connected to motherhood." Morning's chapter focuses on the role of ambivalence in the construction of maternal subjectivity.

Section Three, "Reframing Pregnancy Loss," contains chapters discussing the disruption pregnancy loss poses to normative life narratives and the knowledge generated from such disruptions. In "Reframing the Devastation and Exclusion Associated with Pregnancy Loss as a Normal and Growth-Enhancing Component of the Physiological Female Continuum," Keren Epstein-Gilboa explores how pregnancy loss can be reframed to assist women to heal after pregnancy loss. Although many feel like a "failure" upon losing a pregnancy, Epstein-Gilboa considers ways of reframing miscarriage as a "treasured rather than a deviant event." She argues that assisting clients to frame their pregnancy losses in the context of systemic issues may facilitate emotional growth. By reframing stories of pregnancy loss, Epstein-Gilboa shows that loss can be reconsidered as part of "normal human experience," potentially mitigating feelings of isolation and personal failure. Similarly, j wallace skelton's "failing" considers the role transphobia plays in fuelling speculations about why miscarriage occurs. Exploring the possibility he has a "failed body," skelton asserts that failure is "inherently part of having a body" and demonstrates how certain goals need to be "shifted" in order to be met. "None of it was a failure," he writes, "the notion of failure is what failed." Emily R.M. Lind's "Fatphobia, Pregnancy Loss, and My Hegemonic Imagination: A Story of Two Abortions" considers the extent to which her decision to terminate two pregnancies in her mid-twenties was informed by social pressure to adhere to a traditional model of family. Having internalized the importance of waiting for the "right time" to have children, Lind concludes that the "right time" is a social fiction embedded in hegemonic dynamics of power, such as fatphobia and white supremacy. She considers the regret she sometimes feels toward her decision to terminate but reframes it as predicated on the assumption of a live birth: "My regret is a form of disavowal, as it denies the possibilities that my pregnancies could have ended in miscarriage or stillbirth ... and that is simply unknowable." Robin Silbergleid's "Missed Miscarriage—*for A*" confronts the limitations of both language and knowledge in her essay on miscarriage. Arguing that miscarriage "is not a single definitive event," Silbergleid asserts that in the context of miscarriage, she has experienced "the failure of traditional narrative forms," since "the process was not linear but circular; my experience existed separate from and tethered to the diagnostic codes used to label it." Silbergleid's essay jumps back and forth through time, and highlights the inadequacies of existing clinical categories for early (missed) miscarriage, which invites readers to consider the notion that the truth is "multiple and between." Likewise, Rachel

O'Donnell's "Full-Term Baby Loss: A How-to Guide for Mothers" offers an alternative chronological recounting of the experience of stillbirth, as her narratives describes multiple events in the past and future all while using the present tense. To that end, she uses second-person narration to describe herself: "Look in the mirror at what you have: a bereaved body living in two times at once. Your pregnant body was two bodies, but now you are less than one." O'Donnell's essay reframes the grammar of pregnancy loss and considers molecular transformation as she looks to dirt and mathematical calculations to find evidence of her lost child. The final essay in this section, "How to Hear a Story: Reflections on the Anniversary of my Rape" is written by Rhobi Jacobs who narrates her memories by offering, "we take experiences of particular pleasure or trauma into our cells ... they transform from physical experience into the stuff of our dreams, our poems, and songs, our beliefs about ourselves, and our agency and our futures ... our stories of loss and transgression exist beyond and apart from the evidentiary dimension of rape or the medical event of miscarriage." In this way, Jacobs reframes pregnancy loss beyond a medical event, and considers loss within a broader context of physical trauma and the desire to heal.

Section Four, "Interrogating the Medicalized Logics of Pregnancy Loss," engages directly with the social implications of medical terminologies and medicalized logics. Elizabeth Heineman's "A Death Certificate, an Autopsy, a Pile of Insurance Claims" explores the inadequacy of clinical guidelines to prevent her son's stillbirth. Calling herself "the homebirthing community's worst nightmare," Heineman contends that her stillbirth "probably would not have occurred had I been receiving hospital care." Reflecting on the social power accorded to medical doctors, she argues that "My midwife made a judgment call. Doctors make judgment calls too. But when their judgment turns out to be wrong, it doesn't call into question the enterprise of hospital birth. When their judgment calls turn out to be wrong, no one blames the mother for having chosen hospital birth." Unique in this collection for her exploration of infertility, Maria Novotny's chapter argues that the medical discourse of infertility reveals an ideological position whereby "to be infertile as a female is to be abnormal." In "Failing Fertility: A Case to

Queer the Rhetoric of Infertility," she finds destigmatizing rhetorical tools within the field of queer phenomenology. She invites both scholars and infertility advocates to embrace "more critical, more queer arguments about the ... expectations of heteronormative infertility." This kind of reflective praxis, Novotny argues, "serves as a productive exercise to ponder why individuals are oriented toward certain cultural desires and affections. This is the new work needed for infertile women to embrace as they grieve their inability to conceive." Her work interrogates the cultural meanings of pregnancy from the perspective of gender, sexuality, and identity. In the final chapter in this section, "A Feminist Perspective on Selective Termination," Brittany Irvine argues for an expanded scope of feminist medical analysis on selective termination, a form of loss currently underexamined in feminist scholarship. Selective termination is the "interruption of the development of a fetus in a multiples pregnancy ... usually [a fetus who is] developing abnormally." Irvine argues that selective termination "complicates the discourse of liminality" for pregnancy loss because the pregnant subject who consents to a selective termination experiences a loss while remaining pregnant. Medical literature describes the terminated fetus as a "papyrus stillborn." Irvine suggests that this presents an opportunity for parents to claim discursive authority over how their loss is named and treated clinically.

The final section, "Memorializing Loss," presents research findings on the commemorative rituals and practices used to mark the loss of pregnancy. Miriam Rose Brooker's "Enacting Acknowledgment, Meaning, and Acceptance: Personal Ceremony and Ritual as Helpful Ways to Engage with Feelings of Loss After Abortion" documents the rituals used by women to mark their experience of abortion as a form of loss. She names ritual as a way "to acknowledge and express ... complex and multilayered responses to abortion." For Brooker, ritual fills a gap left by the cultural taboos forbidding talking about abortion in nuanced ways. Similarly, Christa Craven and Elizabeth Peel's "Queering Reproductive Loss: Exploring Grief and Memorialization" argues that creative memorialization practices offer a way of challenging heteronormative ideas about family formation. Situating queer communities as possessing "a long history of memorializing loss," they argue that reproductive loss is excluded in this long history, in part because the history of queer memorialization speaks directly to the "pain and shame of the closet." In their study of how queer families have commemorated the loss of pregnancy and family planning, Craven and Peel show that creative memorialization represents "a beginning for many LGBTQ families, not merely the end." By commemorating loss, queer families incorporate "grief, sorrow, longing, and loss" into conceptualizations of reproductive futurity, and these interventions "have the potential to destabilize 'success' narratives.'" Craven and Peel's findings echo the insistence of many pregnancy loss scholars who argue that linear narratives of reproduction are normative and, therefore, exclusionary to the diversity of experience of pregnancy and parenthood.

The normative and exclusionary constructions of pregnancy, loss, and subjectivity caused the epistemic friction inspiring this collection. When contending with the social significance of our personal experiences of pregnancy loss, we sought out creative and intellectual interventions facilitating new ways of thinking about pregnancy loss. We solicited contributions that made room for an understanding of loss as complex, nuanced, and multifaceted. The seventeen chapters in this collection are the consequences of our seeking. Collectively, they contend with pregnancy loss as a phenomenon many of us confront without adequate preparation. This collection has been compiled to offer a broad range of voices interested in the following: breaking the silence about the nature and experience of pregnancy loss; strengthening an understanding of pregnancy as a relational state of being; reframing the social meaning of loss to access self-actualization; interrogating medical logics that can delineate the interpretive scope of pregnancy and its loss; and finally, memorializing loss in an effort to understand the future as one made possible by past losses.

A NOTE ON LANGUAGE

By interrogating pregnancy loss, the gendered politics at stake in pregnancy were likewise interrogated. This introduction was written with the understanding that not all women get pregnant and that not all pregnant people identify as women. To that end, this introduction has used gender-neutral language to describe subjects who experience the loss of their own physical pregnancies. This rhetorical practice reflects an orientation to gender as socially constructed and trans-inclusive.

In this essay, when citing sources that describe pregnant subjects, I have left the author's gender-specific language (often "woman" or "mother") as it was originally printed. This decision reflects the fact that gender-specific language is a convention in the field of motherhood studies, and many advocate for the sustained use of the term "motherhood" to appropriately highlight the distinctly gendered forms of labour, kinship, and praxis that the term reflects. As editors, we have accepted our contributors' choices to frame pregnancy and the literature that examines it at their own discretion. We invite our readers to experience the inconsistencies, frustrations, and interruptions our editorial decisions have created as reminders of the messy inadequacies offered by both gender and language.

ENDNOTE

[1]Earle et al. define "reproductive loss" as a category that includes abortion, miscarriage, stillbirth, but also infertility, infant death, maternal death, and other losses to normative experiences with reproduction broadly defined.

WORKS CITED

Cacciatore, J., and S. Bushfield. "Stillbirth: A Sociopolitical Issue." *Affilia*, vol. 23, 2008, pp. 378-87.

Cosgrove, Lisa. "The Aftermath of Pregnancy Loss: A Feminist Critique of the Literature and Implications for Treatment." *Women & Therapy*, vol. 27, no. 3-4, 2004, pp. 107-22.

Davidson, Deborah, and Gayle Letherby. "Griefwork Online: Perinatal Loss, Lifecourse Disruption and Online Support." *Human Fertility* vol. 17, no. 3, 2014, pp. 214-17.

Davidson, Deborah, and Helena Stahls. "Maternal Grief: Creating an Environment for Dialogue." *Journal of the Motherhood Initiative for Research and Community Involvement*, vol. 1, no.

2, 2010, pp. 16-25.

Earle, Sarah, and Gayle Letherby. "Conceiving Time? Women Who Do or Do Not Conceive." *Sociology of Health and Illness,* vol. 29, no. 2, 2007, pp. 233-50.

Earle, Sarah, et al. "The Social Dimensions of Reproductive Loss." *Practising Midwife,* vol. 10, no. 6, 2007, pp. 28-34.

Earle, Sarah, et al. "Conceptualizing Reproductive Loss: Implications For Understanding Human Fertility." *Human Fertility,* vol. 11, no. 4, 2008, pp. 259-262.

Earle, Sarah, et al., editors. *Understanding Reproductive Loss: Perspectives on Life, Death and Fertility.* Routledge, 2012.

Gerber-Epstein, Paula, Ronit D. Leichtentritt, and Yael Benyamini. "The Experience of Miscarriage in First Pregnancy: Women's Voices." *Death Studies,* vol. 33, no. 1, 2009, pp. 1-29.

Hudson, Kirsten. "Taste My Sorrow." *Performance Research: A Journal of the Performing Arts,* vol. 19, no. 1, 2014, pp. 41-51.

Hurst, Rachel A.J. "What Might We Learn From Heartache? Loss, Loneliness, and Pedagogy." *Feminist Teacher,* vol. 20, no. 1, 2009, pp. 31-41.

Layne, Linda "Breaking the Silence: An Agenda for a Feminist Discourse of Pregnancy Loss." *Feminist Studies* Summer, vol. 23, no. 2, 1997, pp. 289-316.

Layne, Linda. *Motherhood Lost: A Feminist Account of Pregnancy Loss in America.* Routledge, 2003.

Layne, Linda. "Unhappy Endings: A Feminist Reappraisal of the Women's Health Movement From the Vantage of Pregnancy Loss." *Social Science and Medicine,* vol. 56, no. 9, 2003, pp. 1881-891.

Letherby Gayle. "The Meanings of Miscarriage." *Women's Studies International Forum,* vol. 16, no. 2, 1993, pp. 165-80.

Letherby, Gayle, and Deborah Davidson. "Embodied Storytelling: Loss and Bereavement, Creative Practices, and Support." *Illness, Crisis & Loss,* vol. 23, no. 4, 2015, pp. 343-60.

Lindemann, Hilde. "Miscarriage and the Stories We Live By." *Journal of Social Philosophy,* vol. 46, no. 1, 2015, pp. 80-90.

Lovell, A. "Some Questions of Identity: Late Miscarriage, Stillbirth, and Perinatal Loss." *Social Science & Medicine,* vol. 17, no. 11, 1983, pp. 755-61.

McLeod, Carolyn. *Self-Trust and Reproductive Autonomy.* The MIT Press, 2002.

Parsons, Kate. "Feminist Reflections on Miscarriage, in Light of Abortion." *International Journal on Feminist Approaches to Bioethics*, vol. 3, no. 1, 2010, pp. 1-22.

Sherwin, Susan. "Abortion Through a Feminist Ethics Lens." *Readings in Health Care Ethics*, 2nd ed., edited by Elizabeth (Boetzkes) Gedge and Wilfrid J. Waluchow, Broadview Press, 2012, pp. 238-48.

Steinbock, Bonnie. "Why Most Abortions Are Not Wrong." *Ethics Issues in Modern Medicine*, 6th ed., edited by Bonnie Steinbock, et al., McGraw Hill, 2003, pp. 471-82.

Thompson, Judith Jarvis. "A Defense of Abortion." *Philosophy and Public Affairs*, vol. 1, no. 1, 1971, pp. 47-66.

Warren, Mary Anne. "On the Moral and Legal Status of Abortion." *Applied Ethics: A Multicultural Approach*, 4th ed., edited by Larry May et al., Prentice Hall, 2006, pp. 516-24.

I. BREAKING THE SILENCE

1.
Communicating Miscarriage

Coping with Loss, Uncertainty, and Self-Imposed Stigma

MASHA SUKOVIC AND MARGIE SERRATO

PROLOGUE: WHAT PRECEDED MASHA'S EXPERIENCE OF MISCARRIAGE

IT NEVER CROSSED MY MIND that I could have a miscarriage. It just wasn't on my list of things to worry about. In my misguided mind, miscarriage was something that happened to daytime soap opera characters—the ones who are pushed down a spiral staircase by a nefarious rival or who unexpectedly fall off a horse while riding around their estate. Until I had my miscarriage, I didn't personally know any women who had had one, so in my mind, miscarriage wasn't something that happened to "real" women. I wasn't aware of the statistics either: more than 20 percent of all known pregnancies end in miscarriage (U.S. National Library of Medicine).

It occurred to me much later—after I could look at my own experience through a critical rather than a purely emotional lens—that women rarely communicate about their experience of miscarriage to other women, which explained my woeful ignorance, as if it were a dark secret never revealed to anyone. In many ways, my experience of miscarriage was akin to experiencing a stigmatized illness—one that I perceived as "a sign of disgrace or discredit, which [set me] apart from others" (Byrne 65) and one that I was ashamed of and reluctant to share with anyone.

I began to speak about this traumatic event in my life and share it with other women in the hope I could contribute to overcoming the stigma of miscarriage. This, in turn, led me to share my experience with my friend and the co-author of this chapter, Margie, in one of the first open conversations I had about my miscarriage, which occurred more than a year after it took place.

THE INSPIRATION FOR THIS CHAPTER

We were silent about our lived experiences of miscarriage for a while, which we see as an unavoidable part of the coping and healing process. However, we now wish to share these, still painful, memories and use them in a threefold way: (1) as sense-making devices; (2) as tools to repair and heal our identities; and (3) as vehicles to communicate our stories to other women and those who care for them.

The ways in which we comprehend and make sense of our miscarriages are both similar and vastly different, which reflects, on a small scale, the myriad ways in which women perceive, grasp the meaning of, and cope with miscarriage. In the remainder of this chapter, each of us provides our own personal experience of miscarriage in an effort to shed more light on individual women's perceptions of miscarriage as a disruption in their personal and gender identities as well as an antithesis to the dominant cultural narratives of uncomplicated fertility and natural motherhood. We examine our individual, autoethnographic responses to these traumatic disruptions by using narrative analysis (Frank), social stigma theory (Bohle; Brouwer; Goffman), David Morris's notion of postmodern illness, and the concept of effortless perfection (Dube; Lipka; Ruane; Travers et al; Wyler; Yee) as lenses through which we seek to understand and address the multitude of women's unique lived experiences following a miscarriage.

MASHA'S EXPERIENCE OF MISCARRIAGE

My miscarriage occurred early, at nine weeks. It came as a complete surprise to me. I wasn't concerned about my pregnancy in the least. I was at a good place in my life and happy in my relationship. My husband had just accepted a very competitive postdoc position at an Ivy League University in upstate New York. I was in Texas, working toward a doctorate in health communication and gender studies and travelling to spend time with my husband whenever possible. We didn't have any trouble getting pregnant. I was strong, healthy, fairly young, and in great physical shape. I was doing boot camp three times a week and running on alternate days. I was seriously considering participating in my first Tough Mudder challenge—a hardcore ten-to-twelve mile obstacle race designed by British Special Forces and touted as "probably the toughest event on the planet."

Even during pregnancy, I was affected by the ideal of "effortless perfection" or the myth that women need to excel at everything we do—work, sports, intellectual endeavours, physical appearance, and life in general—without any apparent effort (Dube; Lipka; Ruane; Travers et al; Wyler; Yee). First described in 2003 by the authors of Duke University's Women's Initiative landmark study, "effortless perfection" pertains to the relentless pressure felt by college women to be "smart, accomplished, fit, beautiful and popular ... without visible effort" (12). However, I argue that this pressure affects not only female undergraduate students but female graduate students and junior faculty members as well, albeit in somewhat different spheres of their lives. As a doctoral student, I was expected to produce excellent academic work, but my own expectations of perfection did not end there. I wanted to have a "perfect," uncomplicated pregnancy experience, stay in "perfect" shape, and go home from the hospital carrying a "perfect" baby in my arms. With this expectation of perfection came a clear sense of cockiness and fearlessness; in my mind, nothing could or would go wrong with this pregnancy. Everything was under control because it had to be in order to successfully maintain the illusion of perfection.

But at my first ultrasound, to which I went alone, I learned the hard truth: the embryo wasn't attached to the yolk sac (the umbilical vesicle), and there was no audible heartbeat. The nurse was visibly upset, her brow furrowed; she was doing her best to sound sympathetic. "I'm really sorry," she said. I didn't fully understand. Did this mean that there wasn't going to be a baby? Did I do something wrong? Was it the boot camp? The running? The late nights spent working on my dissertation? My arrogance? How could I have messed up so badly? All of those questions were replaced with one thought in my mind: "Don't let this stranger see you cry." I waved my hand at her in a nonchalant, breezy gesture, my face contorted into a mockery of a smile. "That's okay," I blurted out nonsensically. But it wasn't okay.

My doctor soon explained the nature of my condition: it was a missed miscarriage. This is also known as the "silent" miscarriage because the typical miscarriage symptoms—such as vaginal bleeding or spotting, heavy cramping, or expulsion of fetal tissue—are absent. The condition is fairly rare; about 1 percent of all pregnancies result in a missed miscarriage. The doctor explained that the embryonic death took place, but the expulsion of the embryo did not occur. Nobody really knows why this happens, but a missed miscarriage is typically caused by chromosomal abnormalities, which prevent the pregnancy from developing ("Miscarriage").

It wasn't anything I did or didn't do, the doctor said. She was a runner herself, with two healthy children, and she was sure exercise had nothing to do with my miscarriage. It wasn't anybody's fault. But I felt, with some certainty, it must have been my fault. I finished my conversation with the doctor, and ran to the warm, stifling safety of my car, where I could finally cry without being seen by anyone. None of it made any sense. I was lost. This was the beginning of my chaos narrative: my hazy, unruly story with no real narrative sequence; a story that defies telling (Frank).

MISCARRIAGE AS A POSTMODERN ILLNESS
AND THE CHAOS NARRATIVE

As Arthur Frank explains, illness calls for stories, which serve to "repair the damage that illness has done to the ill person's sense of where she is in life, and where she may be going. Stories are a way of redrawing maps and finding new destinations" (53). For me, miscarriage was very much like an illness: a painful, identity-altering experience that I needed to suffer through and could ultimately recover from. This notion of miscarriage as an illness of sorts further corresponds to Morris's view of postmodern illness as a mental, emotional, and corporal phenomenon occurring at the intersection of biology and culture. As Morris suggests, "Postmodern illness is fundamentally biocultural—always biological and always cultural—situated at the crossroads of biology and culture" (71). In that sense, illness is a product of our socially and culturally constructed fears and perceived inadequacies, which essentially arises from our continuous longing for perfection.

Following the diagnosis of a missed miscarriage, I felt that my body had failed me—similar to the way that a person diagnosed with a severe illness may feel. Moreover, my body had failed not only me but also my husband and my family, causing grief and disappointment to all. It so happened that my beloved uncle had died only three days before I announced my pregnancy to my family members. This pregnancy was like a special boon bestowed onto the grieving family as a replacement for a lost loved one. I was overwhelmed with the burden of guilt for disappointing my family's expectations; the blessing was revoked and the fault was on me.

In a culture that puts such a strong pressure on young women to achieve "effortless perfection" (Dube; Lipka; Ruane; Travers et al; Wyler; Yee), which includes producing "perfect" babies, un-complicated fertility and natural motherhood are not just expected but taken for granted, and are often perceived as the norm rather than the fortunate exception. Therefore, similar to an experience of a stigmatizing illness, an inability to fulfill those cultural ex-pectations can lead to perceived social stigma, self-stigmatization, and, potentially, even an identity crisis (Bohle; Brouwer; Goffman). Moreover, the idea of a "perfect" body is further informed by the notion of whiteness as an invisible ideal in American society. In other words, for a white, educated, and relatively affluent woman, the "effortless," invisible expectation of a successful pregnancy serve, in part, to perform, reproduce, and reinforce the codes of whiteness by providing a locus of cultural performance dependent on whiteness as an invisible ideal.

For me, the miscarriage was a deeply unsettling experience, one strewn with guilt, shame, fear, irrationality, and uncertainty. There is little coherence to my memories immediately following the missed (silent) miscarriage diagnosis. I do remember some of the health choices I made—such as refusing a suction dilation and curettage to remove any remaining embryonic tissue that had not been naturally passed. Instead, I opted for the medical therapy using oral misoprostol, a drug that induces uterine contractions, as a less invasive alternative to the surgical procedure. I told my doctor that this sounded like a better option to me because I wanted to give my body a chance to expel the pregnancy tissue naturally. What I never mentioned to her, or anyone else, was my irrational hope that somehow I could will my embryo back to life in the weeks preceding the misoprostol treatment. My chaos could not be shared or told; it could only be lived in silence, much like the "silent miscarriage" my body was ineffectively grappling with.

I chose to be alone when I finally took the misoprostol. I suffered and bled in the silence of my darkened bedroom. I desperately clung to the notion of my body as monadic, or isolated, from all the other people in my life, and I refused to share my pain and my deep sadness with anyone. As Frank elucidates, "This monadic orientation contributes to the inability to find recognition or support for the body's pain and suffering" (102).

It took me almost three years, and the birth of a healthy daughter, to be able to finally tell my story. I needed the time and the distance to process my own feelings and make sense of them, and to find the strength to revisit those dark, chaotic moments in my life. As Frank explains,

> The teller of chaos stories is, preeminently, the wounded storyteller, but those who are truly *living* the chaos cannot tell in words. To turn the chaos into a verbal story is to have some reflective grasp of it. The chaos that can be told in story is already taking place at a distance as is being reflected on retrospectively. For a person to gain such a reflective grasp of her own life, distance is a prerequisite. (98, emphasis in original)

Moreover, I could not tell this story before in part because the experiences of chaos often "erect a wall around the teller that prevents her from being assisted or comforted" (Frank 102). Now that the wall has been torn down and I am no longer silent, this story, as chaotic and disruptive as it may be, has allowed me to cultivate a sense of peace within myself.

MARGIE'S EXPERIENCES OF MISCARRIAGE

First Miscarriage: Shock and Fear

I miscarried shortly before boarding a sixteen-hour return flight to Australia in a bathroom at the United Club lounge in the Los Angeles airport. There were no symptoms to warn me. There was no pain before, during, or after it happened. There was just a pool of blood, followed by shock and fear. For a brief moment, there was also denial. After all, my only exposure to miscarriage was through television and movies showing the woman waking up in the middle of the night in pain and blood-soaked sheets.

This was my first pregnancy. I barely had two weeks to feel any symptoms and celebrate the surprising but welcome news with my husband and our family. I had taken an at-home pregnancy test while visiting my parents and siblings several days before; the news immediately became public, after my dad and brother posted about it on their Facebook pages faster than the two lines had appeared on the stick. I felt so fortunate—and fertile!—to have conceived within a few weeks of trying. I was relieved to be pregnant because I long had a premonition that something would go wrong. Upon realizing that I miscarried, I first thought how everyone would be disappointed. Before I knew it, the source of our happiness was flushed down the toilet.

I exited the bathroom and approached my husband. He immediately knew that something was wrong upon seeing that all colour had drained from my face. He grabbed my hand as I explained what happened, and we proceeded to hastily pull out our laptops and search the Internet for "bleeding during pregnancy." He attempted to comfort me after reading that a little bleeding is normal. But I knew this was not a little bleeding. I wanted to believe him, so I chose denial for the moment. Alas, the return flight gave me too much time to think about how sad and frightened I felt, especially given the newborn baby in the aisle next to ours. In my heart and mind, I knew I had miscarried.

I tried to understand why this happened. Was it the glass of red wine I drank a few days ago? Did I drink too much coffee? Was it the Excedrin tablet I took to get rid of my migraine? Was it because I had been on birth control for the majority of my reproductive life (for a total of thirteen years)? Was it because of my "advanced maternal age" of thirty-five years? Did my premonition become a self-fulfilling prophecy? Did my worry cause me to stress, and then the stress caused the miscarriage? I wanted to gain some control over the situation or even to assume responsibility for the miscarriage, but the cause of the loss—as I now know well—is entirely unknown and probably unrelated to any of these factors. The futile exercise in wanting to know the cause, in wrongly attributing the miscarriage to irrelevant factors, and in assuming responsibility for it, all leads to unnecessary feelings of guilt because of the erroneous belief that miscarriage is a rare event (Bardos et al. 1315).

The days following our return to Australia were miserable; a follow-up home pregnancy test yielded a negative result as fast as it had yielded a positive result a week earlier. First miscarriage confirmed. The subsequent weeks were equally miserable, as I avoided pregnancy questions from my mother-in-law or just avoided communicating with our family altogether. I felt lonely. Part of the loneliness stemmed from being on the other side of the world in a new country where I had no friends to talk to. Part of the loneliness was self-inflicted because I avoided talking to our loved ones. But another part of the loneliness stemmed from feeling like I was the only woman who this had happened to.

I was sad for myself and angry that I should have to suffer more in life, given my history as a victim of various types of abuse. I was sad for my husband and apologized to him because I felt responsible for the loss—after all, it was my broken body that spontaneously ended our would-be child. He reassured me that no one was to blame for what happened. Then I tried to stay positive for both of our sakes. I kept thinking "If it's meant to be, it will be. We want a healthy baby, so for whatever reason, that fertilized egg was just not right, ready, or developed." I reframed my earlier feeling about my broken body and accepted my body was working just fine. If the embryo was rejected, then something was wrong with it. I was thankful that we did not have much time to get attached to the idea of being pregnant. I was trying to find a satisfactory explanation and a positive mindset that would prevent me from grasping too tightly to the negative possibilities (like infertility) and from lingering too long on the loss.

However, I was greatly distressed to give the bad news to our parents, who had been so happy with the pregnancy of their first grandchild that they told everyone they knew. I was especially sad for my mother-in-law, whose mother had passed away the month before and who told me—at her mother's grave—she was sad about losing her mom, but our baby was sent by God in her place. I felt like a coward because I could not confront them with the loss. I was angry at our family for sharing the good news with others because now they would have to go and report the bad news. I did not want anyone to know that I miscarried. I did not want to talk about the loss. I just wanted it all to go away. A month passed before I told anyone in our family.

I began by confessing what happened to my sister. I was ashamed about the miscarriage. I explained that I did not call our parents because I did not want to lie to them if they asked about the pregnancy. My husband and I had decided to wait until I was pregnant again—to break the bad news with the good news—because we learned that women are more fertile in the few months following a miscarriage. I hoped that was the case because I did not want to wait much longer in keeping the news, especially since my mother-in-law kept asking how I was feeling and when I was going to the doctor. But after several additional weeks of constant questions and concerns about what must have seemed to her like carelessness or irresponsibility for not seeking a medical check-up, I told my mother-in-law about the loss and then the rest of our family. Everyone reassured me they were not disappointed, and their main concern was my wellbeing. Nevertheless, my disappointment lingered, as did the fear of a subsequent loss.

Second Miscarriage: (Un)certainty

Two months after the miscarriage, I felt the same symptoms of pregnancy as before, and my menstrual cycle was late. I knew that I was pregnant, but I was afraid to take an at-home pregnancy test because I would be too tempted to share the good news before the first trimester was over—a mistake that I did not want to repeat. Once again, I miscarried without any warning symptoms. This time, the uncertainty lingered because the pregnancy had not been confirmed with a test. At the same time, the loss was not "official," which meant I didn't have to tell anyone what happened. After counting the days from my previous cycle to this miscarriage, I learned something dreadful: both miscarriages occurred on exactly the same day in the pregnancy.

Third Miscarriage: Pain and Anger

I miscarried again one month later. I had confirmed this pregnancy with at-home pregnancy test. Given what I had learned about the previous two miscarriages, I was anxious as the "Dreaded Day" approached. The entire day I tried remaining calm and positive, and attributed the other two losses as an unfortunate coincidence not likely to be repeated. Then I had some spotting in the afternoon, which understandably concerned me. The bulk of the loss took place as I was sitting on the toilet, getting ready for bed.

The three losses accumulated in my mind and exploded into desperate and prolonged sobbing in my husband's arms; the individual losses were disconcerting, but their cumulative effect ignited an internal chaos. The heavy cramps on the following day reminded me of the loss taking place and the past losses; they were like a physiological manifestation of my mental and emotional turmoil. In the afternoon, I underwent an ultrasound and then a transvaginal scan at the suggestion of my doctor to make sure that my uterus was clear of any remaining tissue from the pregnancy. The technician conducting the procedures could either not say much because of medical liability or simply had no idea what to say given the circumstance. As my husband put it, "she had no bedside manners." A few times she just said "no, there's definitely no pregnancy" or "the pregnancy is gone." Not exactly kind or sensitive wording, but she got the point across. She did not talk through the procedure to explain what was happening, and she did not give us answers when we asked. She just kept repeating: "your doctor will talk to you about it." That lack of information was frightening. Moreover, undergoing procedures usually reserved for checking on pregnancy and life instead of emptiness was deeply saddening. What began as heavy cramps in the morning developed into painful cramps by the afternoon, and they were significantly worse after the ultrasound—largely owing to the pressure of the technician's hands and the ultrasound machine. I felt drained, even throughout my legs. I was tired. I still had minor pain the next day.

I could not understand what could be wrong with me and my body. After all, I lead a healthy lifestyle: we buy local and organic food, we cook and bake from scratch, I am a runner and a strength trainer and was in optimal physical condition, I do not smoke, I rarely drink alcohol, and I never get sick. All of my healthy choices, my remarkable immune system, and the abundance of children born to females in my family (which I expected meant I shared optimal fertile genes) were supposed to *ensure* the ideal environment for growing and birthing a healthy baby. Over and over, I repeated to myself that I was healthy and young and smart and I ate well and I exercised and I was a good person, and how this was not. fucking. fair! Amid tears, at the peak of my internal and external chaos, I complained to my husband about this un-fairness and blurted: "Crack whores can have babies. Why can't I?!"—a complaint not singular to me, as healthy women who consider themselves in optimal health, thus presumably ripe for conception, often compare themselves to whom they perceive as being unhealthy, mentally or physically. Afterward, I felt like a brat thinking that way, but I was sad, disappointed, and angry. There was no one and nothing to blame.

In the grand scheme of things, I was still a healthy, privileged, and educated person with too much to be thankful for. What I said before still rung true: if it was not going to be a healthy baby, then I needed to be okay with it, and I needed to trust my body. I tried to be thankful these losses took place early in the pregnancy and not later. I was trying hard to keep it together for my husband's sake and for mine. Perhaps because we expected this pregnancy to go well and perhaps to keep me positive, my husband talked more about our future with kids. I thought it would not be fair for him to forego having children because of me. Despite my best attempts, I was not doing so well after this third loss. But I fooled myself into thinking I had accepted my miscarriages and was ready to move on.

Recovering from Losses: Seeking Answers and Breaking the Silence

My husband and I continued to search the Internet and medical journals for elusive answers to the recurrent losses. We learned early miscarriages (which occur within twelve weeks of gestation) are common: statistics suggest up to one in four women experience them and most women who miscarry go on to have normal pregnancies afterward ("Miscarriage"). We also learned a few interesting and dismaying things. No one knows why early miscarriages occur and how to prevent them. Even the most ideal environments, like the one I believed I had, do not guarantee healthy embryos, healthy implantations, or healthy developments. Without a cause for miscarriage, anxiety is significantly higher, lasts longer, and has lasting negative effects into subsequent pregnancies (Bardos et al. 1314)—a fact I can attest to and would claim has cumulative negative effects. Moreover, the acceptance phase of experiencing grief can be compromised when the cause of the loss remains unknown.

We learned that multiple miscarriages were not unusual, as statistics suggest that one in ten women experience multiple losses ("Miscarriage"). We learned that fertility plays a cruel role in this matter: women who are very fertile are more likely to experience miscarriages because their "super-receptive" bodies accept all embryos regardless of quality (Weimar et al.). Thus, conception for such women is easy and indiscriminate, and not rejected until later—presenting a clinical pregnancy followed by miscarriage. Also dismaying is that miscarriages are so common doctors will not conduct genetic testing until after three consecutive miscarriages (known as recurrent miscarriage), and sometimes not even then if they are early miscarriages, even though between 1 and 2 percent of couples experience recurrent miscarriages (Weimar et al.). Fearing infertility as a possible result of the multiple losses, I found this news unsettling.

I was desperate to talk to someone who could understand what I was enduring. I did not want to be pitied; I simply wanted to communicate my experience and my feelings with someone who could understand the embodied chaos I was undergoing (Frank 102). Although support is available, many women do not realize they probably know someone who shares a common loss—and publicly discussing your emotions and fears with strangers can be a daunting task. We feel alone in the process because pregnancy loss is not an open topic of conversation. Despite the commonness of miscarriage, "it remains shrouded in shame and silence, even among friends and family" (Bardos et al. 1313). We feel broken, at least temporarily. But we also fear being permanently broken, and the uncertainty of that prospect is haunting. We feel that our badge of womanhood has not been earned. We stigmatize ourselves before someone else does.

My heritage had a severe impact on my distress in relation to fertility because Latinas are largely socialized into accepting that our main role and goal in life is as breeders—an ideology greatly influenced by the concept of *marianismo*, or the ideal of being nurturing and caring characterized by hyperfeminine behaviour (Gil and Vasquez). Although I have actively resisted such archaic notions over the course of my life, the indoctrination was already deeply rooted. In an odd way, learning about "super-fertile" women allowed me to cling onto the idea that I was not a broken link in a long line of fertile women. Thus, it was not surprising to learn that Hispanics are more than twice as likely to believe that miscarriage is not a result of genetic abnormalities (Bardos et al. 1315) because that would negate, or at least question, our ability to fulfill the limited role we have as women. In American society, some of the added stigma from perceived failure is in relation to the women's health movement of the 1970s and the idea that women should, and can, control their own bodies as well as positive birth outcomes: "Therefore, if the pregnancy fails, the implication is that the mother has somehow failed as a woman" (Harris 27). We also blame ourselves because there is no one else whom we can blame and, in part, because our language dictates that we accept wrongdoing.

Language is important in communicating and understanding our world, and it greatly influences our perceptions (Whorf). Linguistically, the prefix "mis" refers to doing something wrong: mistake, misplace, misspell, misuse. The impact of the statement "I miscarried" infers that the "carrier" did something wrong (Lenkinski). Thus, in part, we blame ourselves because of a linguistic inability to communicate about our loss in a guilt-free way. More alarming is the medical terminology used to refer to such a loss: spontaneous abortion. Even worse, when recurring miscarriages take place, the woman is labelled a "habitual aborter." The negative connotation of the word "abortion," which literally refers to the ending of a pregnancy, assumes an active decision-making process; it faults the woman for a loss she had no control over. Both in common parlance and in medical contexts, the words we use have a negative impact on how we internalize and perceive pregnancy loss.

Once I realized that I had no control over the miscarriages, I confronted the loss by talking about it instead of letting silence consume me. When I did that, a terrible and wonderful thing happened: I learned that nearly every woman with whom I talked had a similar experience or knew someone who had. Then, I could believe the statistics. *Instead of feeling like an anomaly, I felt normal.* Upon discussing my losses, the commonness of the experience became real to me. I made it my mission to share my experience so that if another woman was frightened by her loss, she could feel less alone and possibly more willing to share her story with someone who would understand her grief. In this way, I was transformed by my experience of miscarriage and gained valuable insight through it. My sorrowful journey had become a quest (Frank 115). Finding meaning after chaos did not diminish my sadness or my sense of loss. Nevertheless, what had first appeared as an interruption in my story, I later came to see as an opening. As Frank explains, "Losses continue to be mourned, but the emphasis is on gains" (128).

A few months later, I conceived again. This time, there was a heartbeat—a visible and audible sign of life I could be hopeful for. And I was hopeful, but I was no less anxious. If anything, the anxiety was heightened because I was further along in the pregnancy and a loss would be more devastating for us. I shared this fear with my sister, and her wisdom and comfort rescued me from my state of misery, as she said: "I understand your anxiety given the previous miscarriages. But you should not let those experiences rob you of the joy of the possibility for this pregnancy." Those words resonated in my mind. But fear still lurked until after my daughter was born, and even after. One week after delivering a healthy baby, unmedicated and without complications as I hoped and planned for, I thought of my losses and cried uncontrollably. Perhaps I reacted this way, in part, out of relief for the child that now graced our lives. But regardless of the successful outcome of this pregnancy, there are still days—and I am certain that this will last for a long time, for different reasons—when I look at her and it feels surreal. I look at her, and I fear I might lose her yet. It is a scary feeling, but I am mindful of enjoying her now. No one knows what the future holds for us, so the best thing we can do is to live fully today.

Miscarriage Revisited

I miscarried again, almost two years after my daughter's birth. My menstrual cycle was ten days late, but this time there were no symptoms whatsoever. I had stopped taking my oral contraceptives the previous month; the "super fertility" was apparently intact. The miscarriage took place on a Friday, only ten minutes before presenting a week-long team project to a hundred people at a major research university in Pittsburgh. I went to pee before the presentation, and there it was! My exact words, which I unintentionally blurted out, were "Fuck me! Again?!" I knew what it was. Unlike before, I was not surprised but utterly annoyed – and soon thereafter I relived the chaos. I immediately called my husband, who was in Ohio; he comforted me, told me he loved me, reassured me we would be okay, and reminded me we have a beautiful daughter who came after the previous losses. I cried that night. But I was still determined to believe (or be fooled?) that my body was working as it should.

I was pregnant again by the following month. The anxiety from experiencing four miscarriages weighed heavily on me until the ninth week when I had my first obstetric appointment. At the appointment, my anxiety peaked when the nurse asked about my medical history: "how many times have you been pregnant?" I did not anticipate the wording of this question. Increasingly, I have become comfortable talking about my multiple miscarriages—the losses. However, thinking about these experiences as pregnancies— expectations of life, and having to answer "six"—was harrowing. Thankfully, the ultrasound provided some comfort as I caught the first glimpse of our new "little sprout," the name I called our daughter's embryo until I was ready to become emotionally attached. It was my coping strategy: I gave the embryos a term of endearment allowing me to refer to them as our seed of life while simultaneously disassociating them from personhood in the event of another loss. My emotional detachment—or, at least, apprehensive emotional attachment—weighed on me heavily. After so many losses, it seems impossible for me to experience the joy of pregnancy in an unbridled way. But guarding my emotions feels as if I am not loving the potential child or enjoying its existence, no matter how I rationalize it. This guilt persisted until the thirteen-week ultrasound when I could see the little sprout growing and developing all of its different body parts, and I gained enough peace of mind to begin addressing it as our baby.

Overall, my apprehension persisted until our encounter with the baby at the twenty-week ultrasound. This baby, whose growth was progressing normally and whose sex we decided to learn in an unexpected moment of excitement during the visit, suddenly filled me with hope. I talked to him. I was relieved when I felt his movements. I imagined our lives with him and imagined calling him by our chosen name, which made his future more real to me. But I was still painfully mindful that nothing is certain, even after birth. Although I feared I would never be truly free of anxiety, at least I had some hope to rescue me from torment. After our son was born, I could finally breathe in peace.

CONCLUSION

Our individual experiences of miscarriage, though different in the manner in which they occurred and how we reacted to them, are nevertheless similar in important ways. To begin with, we both contended with the illusion of our bodies as monadic. We have both considered ourselves strong, unbreakable women in the physical, mental, and emotional sense. We were both trapped in the delusion of effortless perfection because we believed that we were in control over the creation of the perfect reproductive environment for our babies to grow in. The belief in an ideal reproductive setting, and toward which our healthy choices were geared, was faulty, but it, nevertheless, led us to question those and other choices to gain understanding about, and control over, why our miscarriages took place. Essentially, we felt the need to blame ourselves for the uncontrollable loss—after all, our bodies were, in a way, responsible for ending the lives we had created and carried. This notion of self-blame and stigmatization for both of us stems not only from the societal stigma associated with miscarriage and the lack of communication about it in the public and private spheres, but also from our focus on perceived "perfection" and the ultimate failure to recognize our own humanity and fully accept our flawed human nature. Rather than acknowledging that we are all imperfect beings and our humanity is grounded in this set of beautiful imperfections, we, as humans in general and women in particular, tend to expect perfection from ourselves and our inherently fallible bodies. We dwell in the paradox and the illusion of our "effortless perfection" as we perform and manifest it for ourselves and the world. At the very least, we endeavour to inhabit and embody our own desire, as women, to fulfill the societal and cultural expectations frequently drenched in impossible standards. For that reason, we both unconsciously viewed our bodies prior to the experience of miscarriage as culturally valued vessels of fertility and reproduction and, therefore, experienced pregnancy loss as a "stigmatizing illness" of sorts. Our own feelings of disappointment—coupled with the guilt for disappointing others and failing the unattainable standards of womanhood and motherhood—added another layer of emotional burden to the unexpected and traumatic losses we endured and continue contending with today.

Ultimately, we entered into this experiential and narrative space alone and in silence. But we are exiting together after sharing our common loss with each other—and now with our readers— and entering new spaces of self-realization and self-acceptance. As Frank illuminates, "Voice is found in the recollection of memories. The storyteller's responsibility is to witness the memory of what happened, and to set this memory right by providing a better example for others to follow" (133). Our newfound perspective is a result of our willingness to communicate and co-create our narratives, which was instrumental in our own healing process, and to recognize our own imperfections as opportunities for growth rather than as limitations or obstacles. Even though we have co-created this shared narrative from a clear place of privilege, as mothers to healthy, happy children, we hope that our story can be helpful to other women who feel alone in what initially may seem like a hopeless journey.

WORKS CITED

"Miscarriage." *American Pregnancy Association*, 2017, american-pregnancy.org/pregnancy-complications/miscarriage/. Accessed 5 Sept. 2017.

Bardos, Jonah, et al. "A National Survey on Public Perceptions of Miscarriage." *Obstetrics & Gynecology*, vol. 125, no. 6, pp. 1313-320.

Bohle, Leah F. *Stigmatization, Discrimination and Illness Experiences among HIV-Seropositive Women in Tanga, Tanzania.* Universitätsverlag Göttingen c/o SUB Göttingen, 2013.

Brouwer, Dan. "The Precarious Visibility Politics of Self Stigmatization: The Case of HIV/AIDS Tattoos." *Text and Performance Quarterly*, vol. 18, no. 2, 1998, pp. 114-36.

Byrne, Peter. "Stigma of Mental Illness and Ways of Diminishing It." *Advances in Psychiatric Treatment*, vol. 6, no. 1, pp. 65-72.

Dube, Kate. "What Feminism Means to Today's Undergraduates." *The Chronicle of Higher Education*, 18 June 2004, pp. B5.

Frank, Arthur W. *The Wounded Storyteller: Body, Illness, and Ethics.* University of Chicago Press, 1995.

Gil, Rosa M., and Carmen I. Vasquez. *The Maria Paradox*. Perigee Trade, 1997.

Harris, Darcy L. *The Experience of Spontaneous Pregnancy Loss in Infertile Women Who Have Conceived with the Assistance of Medical Intervention.* Union Institute and University, 2008.

Lenkinski, Ori J. "The Miswording of Miscarriage." *HuffPost Women*, 2017, www.huffingtonpost.com/ori-j-lenkinski/the-miswording-of-miscarriage_b_9067358.html. Accessed 5 Sept. 2017.

Lipka, Sara. "High Court Expands Protections of Title IX." *The Chronicle of Higher Education*, 8 Apr. 2005, pp. A1-A36.

Morris, David. *Illness and Culture in the Postmodern Age.* University of California Press, 2000.

Ruane, Isabel. "Effortless Perfection." *Harvard Magazine*, July-Aug. 2012, pp. 55-6.

Tough Mudder. *Tough Mudder*. www.toughmudder.com. Accessed 11 Jan. 2015.

U.S. National Library of Medicine. "Miscarriage." *MedlinePlus Medical Encyclopedia*, 2017, www.nlm.nih.gov/medlineplus/ency/article/001488.htm. Accessed 5 Sept. 2017.

Weimar, Charlotte H.E., et al. "Endometrial Stromal Cells of Women with Recurrent Miscarriage Fail to Discriminate between High- and Low-Quality Human Embryos." *PLOS ONE*, vol. 7, no. 7, 2012, doi: 10.1371/journal.pone.0041424.

Whorf, Benjamin L. "Science and Linguistics." *Language, Thought, and Reality: Selected Writings of Benjamin Lee Whorf*, edited by John B. Carroll, MIT Press, 1956, pp. 207-19.

Women's Initiative Duke University. *The Steering Committee's Report, 2003*, universitywomen.stanford.edu/reports/WomensInitiativeReport.pdf. Accessed 12 Sept. 2017.

Wyler, Liana. "Variations on 'Effortless Perfection.'" *The Chronicle*, www.dukechronicle.com/article/2003/12/variations-effortless-perfection. Accessed 13 Sept. 2015.

Yee, Cindy. "Committee Unveils Women's Initiative Report." *The Chronicle*, www.dukechronicle.com/article/2003/09/committee-unveils-womens-initiative-report. Accessed 12 Sept. 2017.

2.
Timeline of a Maternal Breakdown

A Feminist Mother's Blog Post
About Her Abortion Experience

ANGIE DEVEAU

My own grief journey feels like a walk up a steep hill.
—Gayle Letherby (135)

I FOUND OUT that I was pregnant the day after Boxing Day in 2013. I was five days late for my period. I was NEVER late. I was also in the throes of parenting a three-year-old boy. I had been suffering from depression and anxiety—a mental challenge resulting from juggling my intensive role as a full-time, stay-at-home mom and working remotely for a feminist maternal academic organization and publishing house. Immediately prior to this time, I started to ignore the strategies and activities I had previously used to combat stress, such as running, weight lifting, and yoga.

When I peed on that stick, I instantly knew I would have an abortion.

Although I loved my son, the postpartum period was less than ideal for me. You know that old saying: "It takes a village to raise a child?" Well, I was still searching for that village. The experience of motherhood felt less like a village and more like a stranded island where I had no hope of being rescued. I often felt alone and had very little support. My husband and I decided very early on that we only wanted one child. We could deal with one.

When I saw that plus sign, I clearly recall how I felt: disappointed and sad. My son was in the bathroom at that time. I remember my husband quickly scurrying him away as I wept on the toilet for what seemed like hours. How could I let this happen? We weren't using birth control. We weren't being safe.

When I called the Morgentaler clinic in Fredericton, New Brunswick, I was six-weeks pregnant. The woman on the other end of the phone scheduled my appointment for the following Tuesday. She told me that the procedure would cost about eight hundred dollars. Ouch! Knowing what I knew about the public system (I spent my final year of my undergraduate degree studying public and private abortion access in New Brunswick, Canada), I could not go through the hoops required for a publicly-funded abortion. The legislation at the time required me to have two doctors certify that my abortion was *medically necessary*. My procedure also had to be performed in a public hospital setting—if my abortion scenario did not fit these criteria, it would not be publicly funded. Although I could not afford the money, I did not want to be judged by my family doctor and be forced to endure horrendously long wait times while I continued to experience excruciating morning sickness.

I was lucky that one of my closest friends worked as a nurse at the abortion clinic. On the morning of my appointment, she picked me up in her car. I remember bursting into tears as soon as I closed the car door. I was utterly terrified. Although I knew that I needed to do this for my own mental health, I did not do well with medical situations in general. For years, I avoided medical professionals because of a debilitating case of "White Coat Syndrome." I delivered my son with the assistance of midwives, so I had not seen a doctor in over four years!

When we entered the clinic, I was very nervous. As I filled out the forms, I remember feeling slightly giddy and joking about some of the questions on the form—perhaps a stage of denial? This stage ended promptly when one woman sitting across from me stood up and ran to the bathroom to vomit loudly. I had not eaten anything that morning, and her sounds were the last thing I wanted to hear as I covered my ears and hummed to myself. Sorry woman. I remember hearing an office staff member ask the woman if she had made arrangements for a ride home with Maritime Bus. This was not the city bus rather an interprovincial bus system, which didn't sound like fun. I was thankful that my house was a mere three-minute drive away.

When I went in for my ultrasound, my nurse friend told me I

had actually measured at seven weeks rather than six. She was a little surprised I wanted to see my fetus in the ultrasound. I had to see him or her so I knew that my pregnancy decision was real. I couldn't think of it as just merely a mass of cells or tissue; a real live person was growing inside of me. This could've been my son's little brother or sister. This was my decision to end a life and I needed this for closure.

After my ultrasound and counselling session—which included a dose of pain reliever and Ativan, an envelope of antibiotics, and the decision to have a copper IUD inserted immediately following the procedure—I sat and I waited for the number four to be called, the number handed to me upon my arrival to the clinic As I waited, a woman with two children arrived and was quickly escorted to a quiet room. This woman clearly did not have childcare or support available during such a stressful time, and I found it profoundly sad. I will never forget the look of despair on her face.

When my number was called, I was escorted inside to another waiting room where I was told to change into my pajamas and a robe I brought from home. After I changed, I sat and waited with two other women—both of whom were mothers themselves. One woman wasn't ready for a second child, and the other had just suffered from a string of debilitating miscarriages and just couldn't go through that awful experience again. We were all terrified. I recall continuously shaking my head and asking myself how the heck I got into this situation. I'm an educated woman. I was sup-posed to know better, right?

When my time came to enter the procedure room, my heart started beating a mile a minute. I became very light-headed as I lay down on the table and placed my legs in the stirrups. When the doctor told me to scoot my bum down to the end of the table, I tried practicing my yoga breathing: breathe in through the nose and breathe out through the nose. This worked well considering I was having nitrous oxide (ironically, laughing gas) during my procedure. When I started to inhale the laughing gas, I didn't experience much physical discomfort, only waves of emotions. I held my friend's hand as the tears poured down my face. I felt great despair and disappointment in myself. I felt sad for the sick woman who had to take the bus, for the woman with the two kids, and for the other two mothers I spoke to in the waiting room. But I also felt extreme gratitude and love—for my friend holding my hand during the procedure, for the doctors performing it, and for the women working at the clinic. A life might have been ending on the table, but these women were saving MY life. The procedure seemed to take forever, although it only lasted about five or ten minutes. Once completed, they performed an ultrasound to make sure that they had taken out all of the tissue and then inserted my IUD. I asked to see the tissue, but it was already gone.

After the procedure, I was escorted into a recovery room, where I was given juice and toast. Once drugs wore off, I could go home. After picking up supplies on my way home, I arrived to the comforting and loving faces of my husband and child. The rest of the day was spent sleeping and recovering. Although the literature given to me stated that some women often felt well enough to return to work immediately following the procedure, I did not. I needed the time to decompress and digest the experience.

The days, weeks, and months following the procedure were challenging. I felt I went through a very serious and emotionally painful experience that many people just didn't understand. I was expected to go back to my normal life and to act like nothing happened. I was supposed to take care of my son and get back to work, but I found this particularly hard. Often the mere sound of my son crying sent me over the edge, and I felt incompetent as a mother and scared to be alone with him. I found great comfort, though, in speaking with friends who confided in me that they also went through the experience of abortion. Many of them lived in complete silence because they feared they would be ostracized for their decision. My depression and anxiety peaked around the second month—likely caused by an imbalance of hormones and a severe iron deficiency, which I found out about the following year.

Following my abortion, I began the initial stages of co-editing this collection on pregnancy loss. Reading through the research, I learned a great deal about the culture of silence permeating society, not only with abortion but with miscarriage and stillbirth as well. I related to Linda Layne's explanation of how the women's health movement emphasizes control over one's body and reproduction, which can contribute to maternal blame when pregnancies do not fit the ideal mold (1881). But not all pregnancies end happily. Although we are constantly bombarded with images of perfect and happily pregnant women with supportive communities and partners, these birth scenarios represent idealistic notions of motherhood and do not provide adequate representations of maternal experience. As Lisa Cosgrove argues, "the vocabulary that health care professionals use to describe reproductive functioning and pregnancy loss reveals assumptions not only about the female body and reproductivity but also about how women who experience pregnancy loss should be 'managed'" (110).

This vocabulary holds merit and has an impact on the encounters of those experiencing loss. Not only did I feel completely alone in my grief, but I felt that as a feminist, I wasn't allowed to grieve. My body, my choice, right?

It has now been over almost four years since my abortion. Since the procedure, my husband has had a vasectomy, and I am forever grateful that I won't have to go through that again. Although I do not regret my decision, I will always have a "what if" in the back of my head. Honestly, I think the "what if" feeling is less my romanticizing the notion of having another child and more my imagining my life and emotions spiraling even further out of control. Following the peak of my anxiety and depression, I decided to begin antidepressants and counselling, which allowed me to come to a point of recovery, acceptance, and self-forgiveness. No one really knows the complete and utter darkness living inside of me at that two-month mark or even in the years after, and no one ever will. But I am sure that the women at the clinic saved my life. And for that, I am eternally grateful.

When I began my recovery, I started a daily yoga practice, which included participating in an energy exchange program where I volunteered my services in exchange for free yoga. I recently watched a documentary on yoga, and one of the speakers talked about the whole notion of karma. They discussed how karma wasn't just this traditional idea that if you do good things, then good things come back to you. It was more about finding and working through your weaknesses and using those experiences to give back to others—it's an action of selfless service. For example, if you have struggled with drug dependency, then once you recover, you should use that experience of recovery to help others in the same situation. This idea really resonated with me. And this is why I have decided to tell my story. I want to help other women who may be going through a similar experience. I want them to know that it is okay to grieve or not to grieve. It is okay to be disappointed in yourself or be depressed, but it's also okay to think that it was merely a mistake and you can move on with your life. Your experience is YOUR experience and it's OKAY!

What's not okay? This culture of silence! I realize a woman's abortion experience is her own, and it is her decision to share it as she wishes. But if she decides to share that experience and needs to do so, then she should have the full support required and not feel judged for her decision. She also needs full and free access to abortion services, both from the point of entry and beyond.

The Morgentaler Clinic in Fredericton closed shortly after my abortion. Another clinic reopened in its place, but private abortions continue to be unfunded in this province. It's disgraceful that New Brunswick does not cover the cost of private abortions; it ignores the basic human rights of its citizens. I fear that by continuing to provide barriers to access, we will continue to see a rise in not only maternal mental health issues but also suicide rates. We must break the silence surrounding abortion so to crush barriers to access, to normalize the experience, and to inform the general public.

One in three women will require an abortion at some point in their lives. She may be a sister, a neighbor, a mother, a friend, or a co-worker. She might need the abortion because she didn't use birth control or because her birth control failed. She might be poor or rich. She might be a teenager or in her thirties (like me). She might experience mental or physical health issues, or she might be the happiest and healthiest person around. That she WANTS and NEEDS an abortion should be the ONLY reason she needs to justify having an abortion. So, let's normalize this reason, so we can move forward and push for needed changes within our healthcare system. I'll go first: my name is Angie Deveau and I HAVE HAD AN ABORTION! If you need to talk about it, please feel free to do so. I am available to listen—with loving and judgment-free support!

This personal essay was originally featured in Stories from the
New Brunswick Abortion Clinic, *by Dammit Janet!*

WORKS CITED

Cosgrove, Lisa. "The Aftermath of Pregnancy Loss: A Feminist
Critique of the Literature and Implications for Treatment."
Women in Therapy, vol. 27, no. 3-4, 2004, pp. 107-22.

Layne, Linda. "Unhappy Endings: A Feminist Reappraisal of the
Women's Health Movement From the Vantage Point of Pregnancy Loss." *Social Science & Medicine*, vol. 56, no.8, 2003,
pp. 1881-891.

Letherby, Gayle. "Bathwater, Babies and Other Losses: A Personal
and Academic Story." *Mortality*, vol. 20, no. 2, 2015, pp. 128-44.

3.
Grief, Shame, and Miscarriage

NANCY GERBER

*We are volcanoes. When we women offer our experience
as our truth, as human truth, all the maps change.*
                                                   —Ursula K. LeGuin

IN HER BOOK *Silences*, Tillie Olsen documents the cultural silencing of women's voices for reasons including (but not limited to) the following: censorship, self-censorship, sexist ideologies prescribing women's submissiveness, the absence of role models, poverty, and racism. Women's stories about their bodies have been particularly silenced because the female body continues to be a site of legal control. In the U.S., women's reproductive rights have recently been attacked through challenges to Roe v. Wade; many individual states have narrowed choices for women (Frankel).

Fears of women's reproductive ability are ancient. Adrienne Rich recounts the story of a Persian myth that predates the Judeo-Christian Bible in which a woman creates the world and gives birth to multiple sons. Fearful that the one who gave them life will also take it away, the sons conspire with each other and kill their mother (110).

Miscarriage—defined by the Mayo Clinic as the spontaneous abortion of a pregnancy before twenty weeks—has long been silenced in U.S. culture. Because miscarriages are frequent—according to the Mayo Clinic, about twenty percent of all pregnancies end in miscarriage—there is a cultural misperception that miscarriage, particularly during the first trimester, is a phenomenon of little emotional significance in a woman's life.

This essay argues women experiencing or expressing grief after miscarriage have been dismissed as hysterical, overly emotional, and irrational. It discusses the role of ritual as well as feminist literary responses affirming grief.

Traditionally, sexist ideologies have equated women with their wombs. The Greek word "*hyster*" means "womb." Hysteria, a condition defined as an uncontrollable outburst of emotion or fear associated with irrationality, was believed to emanate from the womb; for many, "hysteria" signaled women's emotional instability and confirmed their inability to hold positions of power. Thus, a woman crying out in pain and grief following miscarriage is often seen as hysterical.

The idea that human reproduction is a natural function humans share with animals also inhibits women from expressing their grief. The insistence on nature (as in, nature will take care of it) obscures female agency, choice, and empowerment (O'Brien 49-50). And just as reproductive technologies question the essential "naturalness" of pregnancy and childbirth, pregnancy loss undermines the stereotype that women's bodies are containers designed by nature to give birth or that "having a baby as a result of pregnancy is as automatically guaranteed as rain in June" (Hey et al. 127).

Patriarchal ideology insists on women's perfect biological adaptation to pregnancy and motherhood. But as Carolyn McLeod notes, "The cultural construction of femininity [is] a characteristic of childbearing women ... to keep that meaning alive, it is important that women maintain a rosy picture of childbearing" (51). Thus, women are often complicit in hiding or silencing their stories of pain and fear of childbirth out of worry they will expose themselves as ill-equipped and inadequate for the demands of motherhood.

Miscarriage reminds us that pregnancy and childbirth are fraught with uncertainties, even for women in excellent health and even in this era of unprecedented medical technology. Miscarriage afflicts women regardless of age, social class, religion, and sexual preference; it reminds us women's bodies are not machines or assembly lines of mass (re)production, and pregnancy does not necessarily guarantee a child will be born.

In the late 1980s, I suffered two miscarriages consecutively: the first at twelve weeks of gestation and the second, which occurred three months after the first, at six weeks. At the time, no support existed for what I had experienced. No one wanted to hear about a bloody, messy event that began inside the privacy of my body, produced nothing, and ended in nothingness. No one around me acknowledged miscarriage as an experience of loss. Instead, everyone viewed it as no big deal, a minor bump on life's journey. Friends and relatives dismissed my experience, and said, "At least you already have a child" or "You'll try again." One person even said, "Stop feeling so sorry for yourself; my neighbor had even more miscarriages than you did," as if miscarriage were some sort of contest.

Such responses made me feel as though I was not entitled to speak the truth of my feelings; in fact, people who knew me were skeptical whether what I felt could be called grief, since, really, what had I lost? Not a baby, certainly. I once sat at a restaurant with a group of women friends, and when I broached the subject of my recent miscarriage, one turned to me and said, "You're lucky; at least you didn't have a stillborn." Such insensitivity reminds us that women often cooperate with patriarchal silencing of women's truths, which renders them invisible and unspeakable.

Truth be told, I did not have words to name my feelings. I did not know I was grieving. I was lost in an inchoate, confused state mirroring what had happened inside my body: the loss of a nameless, formless mass that would never grow into a living being. I had been an expectant mother, full of hope for the future. After the miscarriage, I was emptied of expectations. If I'd not had another child, would I even be called a mother? In her poem "The Mother," Gwendolyn Brooks writes, "Abortions will not let you forget / You remember the children you got that you did not get." I would add that miscarriage also never lets you forget.

The first time I miscarried, I was at home when terrible cramps drove me into the bathroom. Pieces of a shattered fetus convulsed out of me into the waiting waters of the white porcelain commode. I watched in shock and terror as the bowl filled with large, purplish clots of tissue, membrane, and blood. I was afraid to telephone for help. My body was on its own irreversible course of expelling this fetus; it did not occur to me to ask a friend to come and comfort me. I was both too afraid and too ashamed of my need and desperation to call friends.

Since what had happened to me was not a medical emergency, it took several hours for my husband to get home from work and take me to the hospital for a D&C (dilation and curettage). Scraped out and empty, I returned home from the hospital to a silence and isolation that erased what had just happened: the bloody remnants in the toilet; the detached aloofness of the hospital resident taking my medical history; the cold, blinding whiteness of the operating room; the loneliness and disorientation of waking up on a surgical ward surrounded by people recovering from serious operations. I had not undergone major surgery. I was merely emptied and sad.

And indeed, where should I have been placed after the D&C? Would the presence of a woman who had just miscarried be too traumatizing to the women on the maternity ward? Should the miscarrying woman be hidden to conceal the shame of her inability to birth an infant? My placement on the surgical ward signified my ambiguous status. I was not like the other patients on the surgery ward, but I was not having a baby, as were the women in maternity.

After a two-month waiting period advised by my doctor, I became pregnant again. At the six-week checkup, the doctor could not hear a heartbeat and sent me to an imaging centre for an ultrasound. I could tell from the way the technician scrutinized the blurry image on the screen something was wrong, although she was not legally allowed to reveal what she knew. When the scan was over, she hurried out of the room and left me alone. I went home and waited for the phone call from the doctor that would tell me what was happening inside my body. I felt as though I were a beach ball being tossed from one medical professional to another. Torn between unrealistic hope and the sinking fear the pregnancy was over, I simply waited.

Several hours later—because, after all, this was not an emergency—the obstetrician phoned and told me no heartbeat had been detected, the fetus was not viable, and I needed a D&C. Dazed and numb, I went back to the hospital. The medical resident taking my information was the very same aloof young man who interviewed me several weeks earlier during my first hospitalization. I reminded him I had met him a few weeks ago. He said he did not remember me, although surely he must have recognized his own handwriting on my chart.

After the second miscarriage I became very depressed. I stared in envy at women with rounded bellies, and wondered what was wrong with my body. I had never considered the possibility that I might not be able to carry another pregnancy full term. I began to fear I would never have another child. I began to hate women who seemed able to hold onto pregnancies with what I perceived, in my despair, as a sense of smugness and entitlement. I resented these women, and I was ashamed of my resentment and bitterness, ashamed I had become a small-minded, jealous bitch. If I stood in the supermarket line next to a woman with a sloping belly, I wanted to turn to her and say, you have no idea just how lucky you are.

My obstetrician-gynaecologist (ob/gyn) told me I should stop trying to get pregnant because I'd certainly miscarry again. He pondered the idea of referring me to a reproductive endocrinologist but ultimately advised against it: the tests I'd undergo were painful and expensive. Another ob/gyn in the very same practice told me to keep trying. "Go ahead, see what happens, you never know," he said, as though my body were a roulette wheel. Neither of these men acknowledged the emotional dimension of miscarriage. Perhaps they were familiar with it and didn't care. More likely they weren't familiar with it and weren't interested in learning more about what their female patients were feeling.

The depression lasted several months after the second miscarriage. I dragged myself through the hours as though I had become separated from my body, as though the rupture in my womb had ruptured my identity. I was a healthy woman who wanted more children. Wasn't childbearing my birthright? Why did my body continue to betray me? I believed in ways I could neither express nor understand that the miscarriages were my fault. I believed any fear or ambivalence I'd ever felt about having a second child had contaminated my womb. I felt ashamed that I thought about the difficulties and challenges of motherhood, and now I was being punished for such thoughts. I kept my feelings to myself; I was afraid they were too shameful to be spoken aloud.

Psychologist Alexandra Kaplan writes that when women are discouraged from or punished for self-expression, they can become depressed. Depression, she writes, can be triggered by emotional loss, the inhibition of anger, and a sense of powerlessness and helplessness (209-10).

When I look back at my experiences of miscarriage and depression, I recognize the triggers Kaplan notes: a self-silencing following my inability to find supportive listeners; anger at the indifference of doctors who viewed miscarriage as meaningless or insignificant or who offered confusing, conflicting advice; and the feeling I had lost my autonomy, of being swept along by forces I did not understand. Too, I was afraid that if I expressed my feelings of sadness and loss, I would be deemed another hysterical woman.

A woman's grief following a miscarriage is seen as an exaggerated, even pathological, response to a minor occurrence. Gail Erlick Robinson, a professor of psychiatry and director of the Women's Mental Health Program at University of Toronto, writes, "Many women have little support for dealing with miscarriage. Health professionals may fail to acknowledge the loss, minimizing the psychological effects.... Even if friends know, they may incorrectly assume that early losses are insignificant as there was no 'real' baby" (170-71). Robinson adds the grief following miscarriage may be intense and similar to that experienced after any other significant loss, thereby constructing miscarriage as an meaningful and traumatic event in a woman's life (170).

Grief and shame. Where do those feelings originate?

Grief is a response to loss.

Shame. A sense of humiliation, embarrassment, inadequacy, or inferiority. To feel like one's body is different from the norm, that one is flawed. To be embarrassed to speak the truth of one's feelings because one is confused about what those feelings are and whether they are valid (McLeod 55). To feel one has failed to live up to certain societal norms that idealize pregnancy and motherhood. The perception one must hide one's feelings because to speak them would invite criticism and mockery of the "hysterical woman." Indeed, the epithet "hysterical woman," in its implied redundancy, reminds us of deep-seated gender biases against women's expression of their feelings, since the counterpart, "hysterical man," is unheard of.

It took me twenty years to write about miscarriage and to realize my grief and shame were exacerbated by social and emotional isolation and the self-silencing of my experience:

"Miscarriage"
In the bathroom
Blood, tissue, membrane
Coursing down my thighs.
Twelve weeks.
Not a life, but something.

My friends next door
Having coffee.
I've just miscarried,
I say,
Cradling the phone.
Sorry, they say
As if I'd broken a tooth.

Barren house,
Silent, alone.
I flush the something
Down the toilet.

That painful day as I miscarried, I flushed my voice, along with the lost fetus, down the drain. The first miscarriage, the one I witnessed, was more frightening than the second, not only because I was further along in the pregnancy, on the cusp of the second trimester, but because when I miscarried into the toilet, I became frightened of my body. This was not normal menstrual blood. This was the blood and tissue and organs of a fetus. The twelve-week fetus has a functioning heart with four chambers, distinct fingers and toes, and kidneys that pass urine. The twelve-week fetus wakes and sleeps.

In researching this chapter, I wondered how much, if anything, has changed since the miscarriages I experienced thirty years ago. I do see signs of change in feminist work that documents the anguish of women who have miscarried; it frames their experience in a social context by exploring how perceptions of miscarriage among medical professionals, friends, and family can be damaging to women. This feminist work calls for counselling and supportive listeners, professional or otherwise "who will give uptake to [a woman's feelings], rather than demand different feelings" (McLeod 55). This is important work because it ruptures silence and enables a space for the voicing of grief.

Miscarriage, too, is surfacing from its lowly medical status to an experience commanding more attention in the medical community. Undoubtedly, this shift is due to the increased presence of female obstetricians who take women's reproductive issues seriously and work to undermine sexism. The Internet has also increased the availability of information and access to women's voices. It is easier now for women to inform themselves via the Internet than it was when I miscarried, when medical knowledge was the purview of (male) doctors who supposedly knew what was best. The Internet also establishes an online community of accessible and powerful women's voices enabling the sharing of experience and minimizing shame and isolation.

A recent Google search on feminist writing on miscarriage led me to a series of essays and poems penned by women about their experiences. Two were particularly striking. In Susan Stewart's poem, "A Language," I recognized my own dashed hopes: "then, the miscarriage, and before that / the months of waiting: like baskets filled / with bright shapes, the imagination / run wild. And then what arrived: / the event that was nothing, a mistaken idea, / a scrap of charred cloth, / the enormous present folding over the future, / like a wave overtaking / a grain of sand." Stewart's image of the charred cloth, an imagined (or perhaps actual) burned baby blanket, evokes cremation and death. The image of the wave as the "present folding over the future" speaks to the death of dreams and expectations, and in its folding and unfolding, also evokes the dead baby's blanket.

In "The Miscarriage," Laine Slatton writes about the death of a hoped for future: "The fetus is not going to be a baby, that is not going to be a toddler, that is not going to be my child that I will love and sometimes hate . . . that will cause me to worry the rest of my life." How brave of Slatton to write of mother hate, ancient as Medea, and to acknowledge the ugly, dark side of love while grieving. Such honesty helps create a supportive, healing community needed by women who have suffered pregnancy loss.

Miscarriage is a hidden experience. No culturally accepted rituals exist to acknowledge pregnancy loss. Deborah Brin writes that rituals serve to mark a moment of transition (124). Our lives are filled with rituals, not always religious, as in, for instance, the reading of bedtime stories to a young child. Brin, who is a rabbi, has created healing rituals for domestic violence, incest, and community-wide tragedies, such as 9/11. Rituals help create closure for unfinished grief and a validation of one's experience (124-25). She describes a ritual she created for parents who had lost a child to stillbirth, which involved a visit to the cemetery where the baby was buried and the reading of letters the parents had written to the child. It occurs to me that writing about miscarriage is a kind of ritual giving form and expression to experience. This essay is a ritual.

The expression of a woman's feelings of grief may be complicated by confusion about the status of the fetus. Since most miscarriages occur during the first trimester, the fetus is not a person existing independently of the mother. Carolyn McLeod writes that "In the minds of others, [a bodily relation to the fetus] barely existed, but in [a woman's] mind the fetus may have become part of her already, which would explain why its death had such a profound effect" (155). McLeod's use of the term "death" seems to raise questions about when life begins. Indeed, many prochoice women, including myself, may worry to insist on miscarriage as a loss to be grieved provides fodder to the prolife movement. However, McLeod's insistence on maternal subjectivity—a pregnant woman is a subject with autonomy rather than the fetus as a subject with rights apart from the mother—is emphatically different from a prolife stance.

Long after my miscarriages occurred, my mother admitted to me she had not forgotten her own miscarriage of more than forty years earlier. I was surprised and deeply moved to hear her tell me she was sorry she could not comfort me afterward as she would have liked. No one had been there to support her when she miscarried; she had no memories or experiences of comfort to draw upon. She grew up in a family in which sons went to college and daughters got married. She feared she would be exhibiting weakness in speaking of events long past, which were seen as unimportant and best forgotten. My own mother was silenced by fear to speak her truth to her daughter, and disavowed her history as though it had never happened. Forty years later, the memories of her sorrow and shame were as fresh to her as they were when she was a young woman.

Yet my mother helped me during our conversation, perhaps more than she realized. After my second miscarriage, she began clipping articles about pregnancy loss from women's magazines, such as *Ladies Home Journal* and *Good Housekeeping*. It turns out that in cases of multiple miscarriages, other medical issues may be involved besides an abnormality in the embryo or fetus. I began to make a list of possible causes, including infection or hormonal imbalance. After seeing an ob/gyn who told me to take my basal temperature—an intervention intended to aid conception, not prevent miscarriage—I finally found a doctor who had written a book about miscarriage. It took more than four months to get an appointment to see him. And after one test, an endometrial biopsy, he determined I was suffering from a shortage of progesterone. I would certainly have had more miscarriages had I not been put on a regimen of progesterone.

After the biopsy, it took more than six months to get pregnant. This had never happened before, and I began to wonder if I was suffering from infertility. Just as the ob/gyn began to discuss with me the possibility of fertility treatments, I discovered I was pregnant. The next nine months passed in a state of heightened anxiety, even though the pregnancy was considered high risk only for the first trimester. With the aid of hormones, I carried the pregnancy full term.

Miscarriage is part of the motherline, the cord of women's stories passed down along the generations. I hope the next generation of women will experience healing and support from feminist work enabling and encouraging women to speak about all aspects of their experience. Adrienne Rich speaks of the motherline as a potent force for transformation: "Until a strong line of love, confirmation, and example stretches from mother to daughter, from woman to woman across the generations, women will still be wandering in the wilderness" (246). Grief will continue to be part of the story for those women mourning lost pregnancies. Perhaps the acceptance and legitimization of grief as an appropriate, acceptable response to the experience of miscarriage will bring an end to the internalization of shame.

WORKS CITED

Brin, Deborah J. "The Use of Rituals in Grieving for a Miscarriage or Stillbirth." *Women & Therapy,* vol. 27, no. 3, 2008, pp. 123-32.

Brooks, Gwendolyn. "The Mother." *Poetry Foundation,* 1963, www.poetryfoundation.org/poems/43309/the-mother-56d2220767a02. Accessed 6 Sept. 2017.

Frankel, Emily. "The Role of Female Legislators in the War on Abortion in the American States." Master's Thesis. Baruch College, City University of New York, 2013.

Gerber, Nancy. "Miscarriage." *hip Mama,* vol. 40, 2008, p. 30

Hey, Valerie, et al. *Hidden Loss: Miscarriage and Ectopic Pregnancy,* 2nd ed. Women's Press, 1996.

Kaplan, Alexandra G. "'The Self-in-Relation': Implications for Depression in Women." *Women's Growth in Connection: Writings from the Stone Center,* edited by

Judith V. Jordan, et al., Norton, 1986, pp. 206-22.

LeGuin, Ursula K. "Bryn Mawr College Commencement Address (1986)." *Serendip Studio,* 2017, serendip.brynmawr.edu/sci_cult/leguin. Accessed 6 Sept. 2017.

McLeod, Carolyn. *Self-Trust and Reproductive Autonomy.* MIT Press, 2002.

Mayo Clinic. "Miscarriage," 2017, www.mayoclinic.org/diseases-conditions/pregnancy-loss-miscarriage/home/ovc-20213664. Accessed 13 Sept. 2017.

O'Brien, Mary. "The Dialectics of Reproduction." *Maternal Theory: Essential Readings,* edited by Andrea O'Reilly, Demeter Press, 2007, pp. 49-87.

Rich, Adrienne. *Of Woman Born: Motherhood as Experience and Institution.* Norton, 1976.

Robinson, Gail Erlick. "Pregnancy Loss." *Best Practice & Research Clinical Obstetrics and Gynecology,* vol. 28, no. 1, 2014, pp. 169-78.

Olsen, Tillie. *Silences.* Feminist Press, 2003.

Slatton, Laine. "The Miscarriage." *Trivia: Voices in Feminism*, 2012, www.triviavoices.com/the-miscarriage.html#.WbC31sah-fIU. Accessed 6 Sept. 2017.

Stewart, Susan. "A Language." *Poetry Foundation*, 2014, www.poetryfoundation.org/poetrymagazine/poems/54824/a-language. Accessed 6 Sept. 2017.

II. PREGNANCY AS RELATIONAL

4.
Believing is Seeing is Believing

Elective Abortion and Visual Closure

MARY THOMPSON

IN 2015, ANTIABORTION ACTIVIST David Daleiden sparked a media frenzy by releasing undercover sting videos seeming to expose abortion providers selling fetal tissue for research. These videos and the resulting media coverage added fuel to the ongoing Congressional effort to defund Planned Parenthood. Warnings preceded most conservative media programs covering Daleiden's videos, and included disparaging remarks about abortion providers and the possibility of Planned Parenthood's duplicity ("Meet the Man"). Although Planned Parenthood does not profit from selling tissue (it does use funds to store and transport donated tissue), nor can it use federal funding for abortion services, the media coverage nevertheless reinforced pernicious attitudes about abortion and providers.

Close on the heels of Daleiden's fabrications, antiabortion lawmakers initiated policy for the handling of fetal tissue. Mike DeWine, governor of Ohio, expressed outrage at the process of sterilizing fetal tissue using steam before disposing of it as medical waste. An NPR news program quoted him as describing the process as "cooked and dumped" (Ludden). In Texas, a new rule requiring fetal remains to be buried or cremated after miscarriages or abortions went into effect in December of 2016. Policy makers boasted the policy is "humane," offers "dignity for unborn infants," and that "the mother needs to be given the opportunity to have a say and be informed with what's happening" (Ludden).

As these examples show, the handling of postabortion fetal tissue is poorly understood due to media depictions informed by antiabortion rhetoric, stereotype, and myth. The stereotype tells the story of disreputable back-alley abortion providers demonstrating wanton disregard for women and fetuses. Conservative media programs privilege stories feeding the suspicion that fetal tissue is mishandled and exploited. In 2011, for example, the abundant coverage of Kermit Gosnell, the Philadelphia physician convicted of involuntary manslaughter in the death of a patient, sensationalized the stereotype of abortionist depravity. As feminist historian Rickie Solinger suggests, the image of the "back-alley abortionist," which rhetorically served to legalize abortion, has been dishonorably co-opted to undermine the authority and reliability of twenty-first-century providers.

The fetus has served antiabortion purposes for several decades now, resulting in important feminist analysis of its role in the fight for reproductive freedom (Balsamo; Casper; Duden; Hartouni; Kissling; Morgan and Michaels; Phelan). Over twenty-five years ago, Rosalind Petchesky's "Fetal Images: The Power of Visual Culture in the Politics of Reproduction" analyzed the manner through which antiabortion groups sought "to make fetal personhood a self-fulfilling prophecy by making the fetus a *public presence*" (264, emphasis in original), and identified the importance of imagery in public policy debates. Antiabortion groups have promoted a mythology of "seeing is believing"—the idea that looking at the fetus (via ultrasound representation or directly) will irrefutably establish its personhood and make abortion morally impossible. Much recent proposed antiabortion legislation reflects the myth that being compelled to view ultrasound imagery promotes bonding (although some might say "shaming") and, thereby, dissuades abortion patients. This strategy marks a shift away from the earlier strategies of Operation Rescue, which used disturbing pictures of tissue to stigmatize and criminalize abortion in the popular imagination. Petchesky's argument arose from a sense that feminists had constructed powerful arguments against distorted and decontextualized misrepresentations of abortion, but they struggled to offer a visual counter-rhetoric: "finding 'positive' images and symbols of abortion hard to imagine, feminists and other prochoice advocates have all too readily ceded the visual terrain" (264). She concluded her essay with a call for feminist analysis of women's experience of ultrasound and pregnancy.

Against antiabortion myths, feminists require strategies fulfilling women's needs for factual information about the fetus as well as the potential need for visual closure following elective abortion. These strategies must not burden or shame women, nor should they presume to generalize women's experiences of abortion. This chapter challenges the beliefs that abortion is always a difficult decision and discussions of aborted tissue are "gruesome" and best avoided. That some women elect to donate postabortion fetal tissue should occasion rethinking these attitudes and, at the very least, prompt the question, "What do abortion patients think about fetal tissue?" In what follows, I explore what feminists can learn from the practice of offering patients the opportunity to see their own postabortion tissue. This practice enables some patients to learn about fetal development and view their own tissue as a counselling and educational tool to counter the dominant (antiabortion) visual rhetoric of fetal representation. To feminists who identify as prochoice, this practice may sound risky (or morbid), so I wish to be clear that my purpose in this chapter is to explore the practice as part of the larger effort to keep abortion safe and legal.

Much feminist scholarship on women, reproduction, and technology reflects a fruitful application of Michel Foucault's analysis of biopower, bodies, and knowledge. I rely on these ideas to consider how the visual rhetoric of fetuses and bonding has become the "knowledge" by which women are invited to understand and give meaning to their experiences of pregnancy and abortion. Therefore, I return to Petchesky's work to consider (1) how she accurately foretold the deployment of fetal imagery; (2) how ultrasound (over)use has become part of women's experience of pregnancy and abortion through its alleged role in "maternal bonding"; and (3) how women do and do not "bond" with fetal images in ways defying both antiabortion and prochoice expectations.

My interest in abortion and fetal representation arises from five years of experience as a patient advocate at private clinics and Planned Parenthood. At one clinic, I worked in the sterilization room preparing instrument packages, checking postabortion tissue, and showing fetal tissue to interested patients. In what follows, my methodology is to analyze the clinic's protocol and literature on fetal development and viewing "product of conception" (POC). At the time, I was a clinic employee and not conducting research, so this project does not include interviews. Rather, I consider observable practices, a patient workbook—*A Guide to Fetal Tissue* (compiled by workers at this clinic and other providers in the Midwest)—and, broadly, their effects. I employ the term "product of conception" (POC) for postabortion tissue including uterine lining, fetal material, and chorionic villae. This chapter argues that allowing women to see their POC and inviting their reflection open a space for what Foucault has termed "subjugated knowledges" of the fetus—including an understanding of its loss.

BABY PICTURES AND MATERNAL BONDING

In "Fetal Images," Petchesky was one of the first feminist critics to contemplate the implications of the then growing use of ultrasound technologies in obstetrical care. She asked, "Why has the impulse to 'see inside' come to dominate ways of knowing about pregnancy and fetuses, and what are the consequences for women's consciousness and reproductive power relations?" (275). Her work revealed that obstetrical ultrasound imaging arose in the context of masculinist visual culture, and, using technology infused with military discourse, created a "panoptics of the womb" (277) that sought to secure medical authority over every stage of pregnancy. Furthermore, the resulting fetocentrism suppresses the maternal body and constructs the fetus as an independent homunculus in an adversarial relationship with its hostile surroundings. As a result, the decontextualized fetus is available for the creation of myth, fantasy, and fetishization.

Petchesky's concerns about fetocentrism, medicalization, militarism, and the suppression of women's bodies are realized in the 2008 text *Obstetric Ultrasound: Artistry in Practice* by John C. Hobbins (doctor of obstetrics and fynecology at the University of Colorado). Hobbins demonstrates an uncritical love for the technology and describes ultrasound images simultaneously as transparent "windows" and complicated texts requiring interpretive "artistry." He writes the following: "much has already been written about the brand new 3D and 4D technology, and some of it has the understandable flavor of bias from individuals naturally caught up in the wonder of the technology. I am no different, and am emotionally hooked on the technology to a point where I will engage in hand-to-hand combat with anyone about to take it away" (149). He goes on to observe: "now [ultrasound] can unroof the innermost secrets of the fetus through two-dimensional and three-dimensional imagery and Doppler waveform analysis" (ix). Petchesky's work accurately predicted this medical love affair with technology for its own sake. Her work also foretold the peripheral status of the mother, who, in this statement, is the "roof" blocking the view of the fetus, whose "secret life" has now gained primacy. The mother, presumably, no longer has any secrets worth pondering.

Hobbins also demonstrates his belief in the power of the technology to promote maternal attachment:

> While many providers have latched onto the concept of maternal attachment as a reason to add 4D to every examination (and some have even used this rationale to justify nonmedical 3D and 4D activities), there are at least as many naysayers who cite a lack of evidence of its merit, and even question its safety in this setting … I think that a minute or two of "warm and fuzzy" 4D ultrasound, offered gratis, at the end of each indicated ultrasound examination, will do wonders for maternal attachment and for patient, family, and operator enjoyment. If done routinely, it just might put the "keepsake industry" out of business. (154)

Ultrasound images are believed to enable attachment and, thereby, encourage good prenatal practices (avoiding cigarette and alcohol consumption, for example). Indeed, ultrasound images have become "baby's first pictures" to be shared with family and friends and not isolated in medical charts (Mitchell; Han). Obstetricians regularly send patients home with copies of second-trimester ultrasound images to share with others, and consumer culture has amplified this trend with the creation of "ultrasound and pregnancy baby albums."

At the same time that ultrasound technology seems to respond to the natural curiosity of parents and family, Hobbins's use to encourage "attachment" suggests the unsettling possibility this connection is socially manufactured. Nevertheless, the political usefulness of this alleged connection is clear. Desirable "maternal attachment" has inspired antiabortion policies mandating ultrasounds and waiting periods (Stabile; Morgan and Michaels; Sanger) and has fueled the myth of postabortion syndrome (Bazelon; "Post-Abortion Politics"). Abortion supporters, however, have strongly debated the significance of the ultrasound as well as the idea of maternal attachment. Lisa Mitchell, for example, wryly notes that for all the importance given to "baby's first picture," after birth, the ultrasound fades into memory like other medical procedures. Furthermore, Julie Roberts in *The Visualized Foetus* observes that bonding and attachment are different things. Attachment is a one-way street, but bonding requires reciprocity. Although the women's health and free birth movements have defended the idea of mother-child bonding, the one-way attachment formed by a pregnant woman looking at an image may not merit the same political response.

Other feminists, though, have argued that the experience of attachment should prompt serious consideration. In her essay "My Womb, The Mosh Pit," Sharon Lehner explores the "reality" her pregnancy took on via ultrasound images. Lehner examines how familiarity with generic conventions of photography and documentary inform the "truth" of the sonogram and leaves women who lose or terminate pregnancies with real feelings of grief. Lehner, who aborted when she learned her pregnancy had serious anomalies, observed how the power invested in images shaped her feelings. Pointing out that some women in her situation choose to give birth to see and grieve their lost child, Lehner explains,

> Do not misunderstand me—I do not argue here that the fetus of the sonogram is, simply the right wing icon: the unborn child. Instead I wish to complicate the relative political silence of the feminist left on the complexity of the fetus, as image and as infant. It is not enough to say, "a fetus is nothing more than an image" and be done with

it. This statement ignores the very history of genre conventions upon with sonograms build their claims to medical fact. Images ARE real, insofar as they offer pleasure, cause pain, and incite viewers to action. (548)

Images, then, inform not only the fraught politics of the fetus but also the personal significance of its loss. The rise of infant bereavement photography, for example, may reflect such feelings (Keane; "Infant Bereavement"). In her essay, Lehner observes that "I bonded with an image, I aborted an image, and I deeply mourn an image" (548). Indeed, Petchesky acknowledged this in her work:

To suggest that the timing of maternal-fetus or maternal-infant attachment is a biological given (for example, at 'quickening' or at birth), or that 'feeling' is somehow more 'natural' than 'seeing,' contradicts women's changing historical experience. On the other hand, to acknowledge that bonding is a historically and culturally shaped process is not to deny its reality. (283)

Furthermore, these feelings of loss are not unique to women having selective abortions; many women experience elective abortion as a loss.

As predicted by Petchesky, a complicated task faces feminists and prochoice supporters as they assess the visual politics of the fetus. On the one hand, they dispute the anthropomorphized and fetishized "unborn child" promoted by antiabortion groups. On the other hand, they seek to honor the sense of connection fostered by ultrasound technology and the loss of connection abortion may produce.

A GUIDE TO FETAL TISSUE AND VIEWING POSTABORTION POC

According to Carol Joffe, good abortion-patient care arises from providers meeting each woman "where she is at" (124). This patient-centred philosophy is reflected in the clinic I write about, which opened in the 1980s and offers first and second-trimester abortions, regular gynecological care, and open-adoption services.

The clinic's original owner was a feminist activist who, in the spirit of the Women's Health Movement, employed her physicians and rejected physician-owned clinics out of the concern they did not put the patient first. Over the years, the clinic has survived repeated antiabortion attacks—including a firebombing and anthrax threats. According to staff, the clinic prioritizes patient care instead of "throwing resources" into community activism—an uncertain strategy that nevertheless attends to patients "where they are at." Staff members point to the example of how the clinic uses the state-mandated, twenty-four-hour waiting period. Rather than conceding to the state's goals for this contact, advocates meet one-on-one with each patient to discuss her decision in depth and beyond the required "informed consent" script. Patients share reactions to the biased, state-mandated literature, seek clarification, and deconstruct the antiabortion messages reflected in these documents. This strategy modestly co-opts the imposed waiting period to encourage women's self-expressions and resistance.

In response to both antiabortion policy and patient interest, the clinic staff created strategies for engaging with the fetus. Although patients were required to receive biased, state-mandated information on fetal development, the clinic made available to interested patients its own in-house publication, *A Guide to Fetal Tissue* ("*A Guide*"). The clinic also instituted a formal protocol for inviting and showing interested patients their own tissue or "POC" (product of conception). Although other clinics engage in this practice (Joffe), none have codified it as thoroughly. In my experience at other clinics, patients requesting to see their tissue were sometimes accommodated but met with skepticism. The clinic I write about makes the opportunity to view fetal tissue available to all patients and implements a carefully developed practice, involving clinic staff and literature.

To be clear, this practice is not forced upon or required of all patients in the manner of state-mandated literature and images. The offer to view fetal development images and POC is made on patient in-take charts. A small number (approximately 10 percent) of patients express interest in the option, whereas an even smaller number actually follow through and view their POC. Furthermore, a patient can decide not to view the images or tissue at any point.

Patient advocates are also trained to screen out women who seem to be forcing themselves to look at the images or punishing themselves by looking at them.

Using *A Guide,* advocates first show an interested patient a hand drawn image of a fetus corresponding to her gestational stage. The drawn picture includes an image of a ruler for perspective and explanations of fetal development. Next the advocate asks the patient if she wants to see photos of POC from *A Guide.* After a verbal description, the advocate will show her photos of tissue in a Pyrex dish on a light box. The POC is divided into uterine lining, chorionic villae, and, if visible, fetal or embryonic tissue. Embryonic tissue is visible as early as eight to ten weeks (measured from the first day of the woman's last normal period), although it will most likely be pulled apart. Advocates do not disguise this fact, but they discuss fetal development and reputable research on fetal sensation with patients.

After being shown *A Guide* and following her abortion, a patient has the option of viewing her POC. The patient is taken to the instrument sterilization room where the POC is prepared in a Pyrex dish on a light-box as depicted in *A Guide.* The POC is separated into uterine lining, chorionic villae, and embryonic or fetal tissue. There is no effort to disguise the fetal tissue or, when it happens, its dismemberment. As I did on numerous occasions, an advocate explains the tissue, asks if the patient has questions, invites her to take her time, and engages her in discussion. Patients spend time talking about what they see and feel; they ask questions about fetal development and disposal (it is sent to a medical waste company for incineration), and they occasionally pray over or address the tissue. The women who opt to view POC typically do so for the following reasons. Some patients work in healthcare and have a professional curiosity. Other patients, concerned about missed abortion (when some POC is not removed thus posing the risk of infection), view tissue to confirm the procedure's success. Most often, patients view POC as a way to find closure.

Patient responses to looking at POC were generally positive. When asked afterwards by advocates (as part of the clinic protocol), few patients expressed regret for having viewed POC. Most patients expressed amazement, wonder, and/or some mild aversion ("Gross" was a common initial reaction). As mentioned earlier, one goal for making POC available is to provide patients with accurate information about fetal development. Interestingly, despite being prepared by *A Guide,* some women were surprised what they saw was bigger *or* smaller than they expected—and they appeared untroubled by these expectations. This reaction reveals a dynamic by which women "toggled" between external sources of information, their observations, and their understanding of those observations. This dynamic of "believing is seeing is believing" appears more complex than a simple top-down model of ideological indoctrination.

Additionally, the protocol for looking at POC did assist some patients in identifying and grieving the loss they experienced from elective abortion. The process opened a dialogue between the advocate and patient about her feelings and successfully put her voice back into the representation of the fetus. For example, one of the important ways the clinic sought to "meet patients where they are at" was through matching their discourse. Although *A Guide* uses medical terminology ("fetus" and "embryo"), the advocates adapted their language to match the patients' words, which often meant referring to "the baby." While showing POC to patients, advocates did not "correct" women's language. This code switching, as Rayna Rapp terms it (82-3), on the part of advocates allowed patients to identify their pregnancy. For some women, their experience of pregnancy—regardless of gestation or desirability—was one of connection to a "baby," which, nevertheless, did not dissuade them from abortion.

As mentioned earlier, patient reactions were as varied as the women: astonishment, relief, wonder, curiosity, and grief. Some women expressed their grief by directly addressing the tissue—either asking for forgiveness, or offering prayers, blessings, apologies, explanations, a wish to be at peace, or to join a deceased family member. Some women also claimed the identity of "mother" in these addresses: "Mommy is sorry, but I needed to do this"; "I love you"; and "Mommy hopes you understand." These soliloquys assert and/or insert a maternal voice into understandings of the fetus and its loss. These moments of direct address reclaim representations of the fetus, its loss, and a disquieting maternal subjectivity.

The equivocal yet powerful dynamic of maternal address to aborted children is captured in literature by Gwendolyn Brooks's well-known poem, "The Mother." Although some readers (mis) interpret the poem as taking an antiabortion position, other readers detect a less certain message. This uncertainty arises from the ambivalent tone of the poem's speaker, a mother who addresses her aborted children:

> If I stole your births and your names, / Your straight baby tears and your games, / Your stilted or lovely loves, your tumults, your marriages, aches, and your deaths, / If I poisoned the beginnings of your breaths, / Believe that even in my deliberateness I was not deliberate. / Though why should I whine, / Whine that the crime was other than mine?— / Since anyhow you are dead. / Or rather, or instead, / You were never made.

In her well-known essay, literary critic Barbara Johnson analyzes Brooks's poem in terms of "apostrophe"—"the direct address of an absent, dead, or inanimate being by a first-person speaker" (694)—to argue traditional lyric poetry's use of the figure reflects a male speaker's desire to animate his subject and his need for the subject to validate him. In the case of Brooks's mother, however, addressing aborted children, apostrophe is disrupted by a splitting of the speaker's voice simultaneously undermining her control as well as the certainty of the child's status (699). Arguing for renewed consideration of the political nature of rhetoric, Johnson concludes that "rhetorical, psychoanalytical and political structures are profoundly implicated in one another. The difficulty in all three would seem to reside in the attempt to achieve full elaboration of any discursive position other than that of child" (706). In her reading of Brooks's poem, Johnson exposes the limited positions from which women having elective abortions can speak to, for, and about the fetus.

MATERNAL VOICES AND SUBJECTIVITIES

Does ultrasound imagery make women's experience of elective

abortion more difficult, more grief inducing? I do not believe it necessarily does. Certainly antiabortion policies intend ultrasounds to overburden and shame women (by requiring screenings, mandating that patients look at images, and requiring waiting periods between screenings and procedures). But what the images mean to women and their experiences of abortion is unclear. What do abortion patients have to tell feminists about the fetus?

To some, viewing POC may seem morbid or appear to risk reinforcing antiabortion visual rhetoric. I do not discount this risk, but I believe it is outweighed by the benefit of having patient-provider honesty, accurate information, and an opportunity to grieve. In my experience, only a few patients expressed regret for having seen POC, and in those cases, the regret was specific to seeing the tissue and not to having the abortion. Patients told me that viewing POC was a relief, informative, and a source of closure. The clinic staff defended the practice. They argued that allowing women to explore feelings about and connections to the fetus, rather than troubling their decisions, assisted them in gaining peace of mind.

Beyond the benefits to the individuals who view their tissue, broader potential exists in the clinic protocol for showing POC. First, this practice counters the antiabortion myths of provider indifference and abuse of fetal tissue. Patients deserve to have their feelings and concerns acknowledged. They deserve to know what happens to fetal tissue (during the procedure and in terms of its disposal) and to have their ability to handle that information trusted. Clinic staff frequently observed the importance of providers not "shielding" (which they perceived as condescending) women from the realities of abortion.

Second, by honorably providing patients with opportunities to grieve, abortion providers are not encouraging false grief or reinforcing the myth of postabortion syndrome. I align myself with Katha Pollitt's unapologetic defense of abortion in her recent work *Pro*, but I disagree with her implication in acknowledging grief, providers and prochoice supporters have somehow conceded to postabortion syndrome. Accepting rather than denying grief and the other attendant complicated feelings around unplanned pregnancy aids some women in having a positive abortion experience and may subsequently encourage them to vote in support of abortion access. Additionally, as the Guttmacher Institute reports, six out of ten abortion patients have children ("Induced Abortion"), and in my clinical experience, these mothers express a complex sense of loss. It seems unlikely that women who have experienced pregnancy and childbirth in addition to abortion are simply dupes of an antiabortion script telling them to grieve.

And finally, this practice defends abortion through fostering women's sense of empowerment and control. All too often women facing unplanned pregnancy do not feel empowered by their choices and instead feel judged and ashamed (Joffe). This is not surprising since women make their decisions about unplanned pregnancies in a cultural context that neither supports nor believes in their abilities to make sound, moral decisions for themselves and their children. Young women, poor women, and women of colour in particular feel the constraints of hostile social attitudes. Prochoice supporters must be careful not to repeat these beliefs about women by assuming they must be shielded either from the reality of aborted tissue or from feelings of loss and grief. Subjective understandings of the fetus can be beneficially addressed by having the option to see POC. For the women who choose to view tissue, the process can create a powerful space for the reinsertion of female/maternal voices and subjectivities into fetal representations.

WORKS CITED

Balsamo, Anne. *Technologies of the Gendered Body: Reading Cyborg Women.* Duke University Press, 1996.

Bazelon, Emily. "Is There a Post-Abortion Syndrome?" *New York Times Magazine*, 21 January 2007, www.nytimes. com/2007/01/21/magazine/21abortion.t.html. Accessed 16 Sept. 2017.

Brooks, Gwendolyn. "The Mother." *The Norton Anthology of African American Literature*, 2nd ed., edited by Henry Louis Gates and Nellie McKay, W.W. Norton and Company, 2001, pp. 1625-26.

Casper, Monica. *The Making of the Unborn Patient: A Social Anatomy of Fetal Surgery.* Rutgers University Press, 1998.

Duden, Barbara. *Disembodying Women.* Harvard University Press, 1993.

Foucault, Michel. *The History of Sexuality: Volume I: An Introduction.* Vintage, 1990.

Han, Sallie. "Seeing Like a Family, Looking Like a Baby: Fetal Ultrasound Imaging." *Pregnancy in Practice: Expectation and Experience in the Contemporary US*, 1st ed., Berghahn Books, 2013, pp. 76-98.

Hartouni, Valerie. "Fetal Exposures." *Camera Obscura*, vol. 10, 1992, pp. 131-49.

Hobbins, John C. *Obstetric Ultrasound: Artistry in Practice.* Blackwell Publishing, 2008.

"Infant Bereavement" and "Testimonials." *Now I Lay Me Down to Sleep*, www.nowilaymedowntosleep.org/. Accessed 27 May 2008.

"Induced Abortion in the United States." *Guttmacher Institute,* Jan. 2017, www.guttmacher.org/fact-sheet/induced-abortion-united-states. Accessed 5 July 2017.

Joffe, Carol. *Dispatches from the Abortion Wars: The Costs of Fanaticism to Doctors, Patients, and the Rest of Us.* Beacon Press, 2009.

Johnson, Barbara. "Apostrophe, Animation, and Abortion." *A World of Difference.* Johns Hopkins University Press, 1987, pp. 184-99.

Keane, Helen. "Foetal Personhood and Representations of the Absent Child in Pregnancy Loss Memorialization." *Feminist Theory*, vol. 10, no. 2, 2009, pp. 153-71.

Kissling, Frances. "Is There Life After Roe? How to Think about the Fetus." *Abortion Under Attack: Women and the Challenges Facing Choice,* edited by Krista Jacob. Seal Press, 2006, pp. 189-206.

Lehner, Sharon. "My Womb the Mosh Pit." *The Feminism and Visual Culture Reader*, edited by Amelia Jones. Routledge, 2002, pp. 545-50.

Ludden, Jennifer. "Lawsuit Challenges Fetal Burial Rule in Texas." *The Two Way: Breaking News from NPR,* 12 Dec 2016, www.npr.org/sections/thetwoway/2016/12/12/505304688/lawsuit-challenges-fetal-burial-rule-in-texas. Accessed 16 Dec. 2016.

"Meet the Man Who Exposed Planned Parenthood." *Fox Nation,*

23 July 2015, http://nation.foxnews.com/2015/07/23/meet-man-who-exposed-planned-parenthood. Accessed 16 Dec. 2016.

Morgan, Lynn, and M. Michaels. *Fetal Subjection, Feminist Positions*. University of Pennsylvania Press, 1990.

Mitchell, Lisa. *Baby's First Picture: Ultrasound and the Politics of Fetal Subjects*. University of Toronto Press, 2001.

Phelan, Peggy. "White Men and Pregnancy: Discovering the Body to be Rescued." *Unmarked: the Politics of Performance*. New York: Routledge, 1993, pp. 130-145.

Petchesky, Rosalind. "Fetal Images: The Power of Visual Culture in the Politics of Reproduction." *Feminist Studies*, vol. 13, no. 2, 1987, pp. 263-92.

Pollitt, Katha. *Pro: Reclaiming Abortion Rights*. Picador, 2014.

"Post-Abortion Politics." *NOW with David Brancaccio*. PBS, 25 July 2007.

Rapp, Rayna. *Testing Women, Testing the Fetus: The Social Impact of Amniocentesis in America*. Routledge, 2000.

Roberts, Julia. *The Visualised Foetus*. Ashgate Publishing Limited, 2012.

Sanger, Carol. "Seeing and Believing: Mandatory Ultrasound and the Path to a Protected Choice." *UCLA Law Review*, vol. 56, 2008, p. 351-408.

Stabile, Carol. "Shooting the Mother: Fetal Photography and the Politics of Disappearance." *Camera Obscura* vo. 10, 1992, pp. 178-205.

Solinger, Rickie. "Justifying Choice: The Back Alley Butcher as Spectral Icon." *Beggars and Choosers: How the Politics of Choice Shapes Adoption, Abortion, and Welfare*. Hill and Wang, 2001, pp. 37-64.

5.
The Ambiguous Space of Motherhood

The Experience of Stillbirth

MAYA E. BHAVE

MOTHERHOOD IS OFTEN UNDERSTOOd as the state of being a mother, or a female parent. What does the space of mothering look like? What happens if you lose a child in utero or near delivery? Are you called a nonmother or postmother after such an event? Such nomenclature seems to defy logic. Women whose infant children have died struggle to reconcile a pregnancy and state of motherhood that does not follow a standard narrative for pregnancy: conception, growth, and birth. With pregnancy loss, the jubilant delivery celebration becomes muted, and the culmination of "new motherhood" is completely transformed and reconstructed, often in silent, painful ways. These women recognize that their motherhood falls within an often-unspoken liminal time and space: their status as mothers is turned upside down and its validity questioned. What constitutes the space of motherhood, therefore, is a critical question to examine within the framework of social science, as the answers affect not only how individuals understand the process of taking care of children but also what it means to mother without any children present or how to continue mothering other living children after the tragic loss of a child.

For many women around the globe, the space of motherhood is ambiguous. The mothers I refer to are those whose infant children have, tragically, died unexpectedly.[1] In this chapter, I examine how the loss of a child affects motherhood, particularly through stillbirth. I bring together two distinct methods to accomplish my task. First, I rely primarily on medical and social science literature written about families who have experienced such losses. Such

76

data allows me to explore how these experiences are framed by both medical practitioners and social scientists. These data show that stillbirths are happening at a dramatic rate, yet they are largely ignored by both medical practitioners and the broader, western academic community. Second, throughout the chapter, I insert my own experience of loss by means of vignettes (in italics), as I recall my very first pregnancy, which resulted in the stillbirth of my son Andrew at forty weeks. This unique framework allows the reader to connect disparate, objective data to rich, intimate, reflections. As the author, I do not claim to speak for all mothers who have been in my situation; instead, I allow the aforementioned broader data to speak to those experiences. The detailed vignettes and retrospection insert into the text a mother's personal thoughts.

I begin by examining how motherhood is conceptualized in the West, and then explore how a stillbirth alters the entire birthing experience resulting in an often bewildering, postbirth adjustment. In considering this new reality, I examine how women struggle with shame and guilt at the individual level, strive awkwardly without their child within the family sphere, and finally wrestle in the public sphere to find a community to listen to their thoughts and constructed narrative. This research exposes how women often grapple with such transformed pregnancies alone and implores us to find better ways to acknowledge discuss stillbirths in the medical profession and in society at large.

THE SPACE OF MOTHERHOOD

From the Western perspective, motherhood is a pivotal social role within the institution of the family, which focuses on tangible assets—children, and their subsequent worth and value within the structural unit. As Ann Crittenden describes women's influence on economic history, "Women were recruited to the crucial task of producing ... human capital" (51). As labour moved from the farm to the factory, women produced "a new domestic product"—children (51).

People thus become valued on the basis of their contributions to others and the broader society during their lives.[2] Crittenden argues that women's roles are to "produce" children, called "worker-citizens," and thus mothering involves a critical role of nurturing, transforming, and developing young lives to become something that will benefit the broader community (51). Contemporary mothers are valued for how they interact with children and for how much physical and emotional care they provide them. Mothers who do not dedicate copious time to their children are judged as unfit mothers.

Grieving mothers of stillborn children, however, fall into an ambiguous space of motherhood in which an expected child is not present. Their mothering of this "nonchild," thus, cannot be measured by the aforementioned standards. In some cases, women lose their firstborn child and are not considered mothers at all. In other cases, women have living children at home but are still classified as being "nonmothers" to their deceased infants. They are grieving their lost potential to be mothers and to show their mothering capabilities. Such a mother is deemed a "nonmother"—a person with less value yet with increased emotional complexity. This awkward combination often leaves grieving mothers socially isolated while they suffer through physical and emotional uncertainty.

In the United States, state and government officials add to this burden by not recognizing the birth of stillborn children. In fact, as of 2016, only thirty-four states acknowledge stillborn children as living entities and issue birth certificates for them (MISS Foundation). Thousands of children in the United States are born but are never documented as having lived; their lives appear unacknowledged and invalidated. A child's worth, then, is only realized in "livedness," in the tangible, reified nature of being. Thus, within the context of mothering, and drawing once again on Ann Crittenden's work, only experience and material existence are valued, not thought, desire, or memory.

This ambiguous space of motherhood, then, is often not mentioned, discussed, or examined within society. Phenomenologists, however, do recognize that such nontangible, nonphysical space exists, even if it is not commonly discussed. Henri Lefebvre argues that in the production of space, "Death must be both represented and rejected. Death too has a 'location,' but that location lies below or above appropriated social space; death is relegated to the infinite realm" (35), which he argues is outside the valued space of social life. Death and social life, therefore, do not intermingle in his analysis.

Lefebvre further argues that "by means of the body ... space is perceived, lived—and produced," (Lefebvre 162), yet he seems to imply a body must have breath in the real world. If we use Lefebvre's framework, then, the space of motherhood cannot be one of potential and hope; it must be, as he describes broad life and production, a "social and mental" space (260). Stillborn children do not enter such a space and, therefore, fall into the amorphous space of lost identity.

THE INITIAL SHOCK

So what of the women who lose infants and are propelled into such amorphous spaces? What are their social mechanisms for dealing with such an unexpected blow? The literature shows women face shock, isolation, and a conspiracy of silence, which does not help their grief process.

G.L. Higgins, director of family medicine at the University of Alberta, notes in his research on family grief that "The death of an infant, clearly a major crisis, has a marked impact on the family and its members. For the mother whose child is stillborn, the birth is not the exciting, rewarding event ... instead there is the bitter futility of the nine months of pregnancy which promised so much and quite literally delivered so little" (1556).

So much of the experience was marked by time. I remember the days and events like they were yesterday. I had started labouring on March 14th, and on the 15th, my water broke, and I headed in to deliver Andrew. To my dismay, they told me my water was intact and "he was fine." They sent me home, yet I felt like they hadn't heard me. March 16th arrived, and I laboured without progression all day. Finally at 6:00 p.m. that same evening, he shuddered and fell silent at 6:00 p.m. By March 17th, I was sure something wasn't right given my pain and discomfort. I frantically made calls

*and arrived with my husband at my obstetrician's office at
11:00 a.m. It was at 11:20 a.m. when my doctor uttered,
"He's gone. I'm so sorry, he's gone." What was she saying?
What is she saying? Her mouth was moving. I looked at
the clock and couldn't speak. The moment was silent.*

THE BEGINNING OF THE ISOLATION

Thus, Higgins argues that there are no happy memories of the birth
experience, only negative ones. He also notes that after women
lose children, the hospital actively works to keep them from the
normal birth experience—separating them in areas away from
other mothers—and often "she is not encouraged to voice her
feelings" (1556).

*I learned later that they had marked my door with a rose
sticker. This let anyone entering the room know that a
baby had died. Later that night, as I was wheeled to the
elevator, we passed through the waiting room. A table was
littered with plastic cups and an empty champagne bottle.
My stomach dropped. I knew there were no celebrations
for stillborn children. No one was raising a glass; they were
only struggling with what to say. The attendant whisked
me away to stay in a room on the surgical floor, noting
that "They didn't want me to have to hear new babies."*

Emanuel Lewis, a British psychiatrist at Charing Cross Hospital
in London, confirms such findings. He notes that medical staff
tend to isolate and avoid the newly bereaved mother; they sometimes discharge her early, hoping to protect her "from the painful
awareness of live babies" (303). Lewis further argues that such
actions actually mean "hospital staff do not have to face their
own anxiety about stillbirth." He says that stillbirth is a common
tragedy, "yet after a stillbirth everyone tends to behave as if it had
not happened" (303).

Lam Suk Yee's work documents the typical reactions to a stillbirth—shock, numbness, denial, shame, guilt, self-blame, anxiety,
sadness, grief, depression, anger, irritability, and restlessness (121).

Yee notes that this pattern is typical, but experiences vary from person to person. Yee's work as a researcher at the Royal Women's Hospital in Australia shows that stillbirth bereavement, however, is unique compared with other types of bereavement because the death "may be sudden and unexpected," and there are no living memories of the deceased (121).

> *As Dr. K determined that Andrew had died, I stared at the clock and my first reaction was "How am I going to tell my parents? What will I say?" Immediately, my husband and the attending physician kept pushing me, "Maya, say something. Say something." I had nothing to say. This just wasn't happening. I quickly recalled the earlier events of the weekend at labour/delivery. I knew I had been right, my water had broken, but they wouldn't listen to me. I started to yell, "I told them. I told them."*

Lewis discusses a "conspiracy of silence," according to which "family, friends, and professionals continue to avoid talking to the bereaved mother, depriving her of the talk that would help her mourn" (303). Jean Stringham et al. note even the medical literature perpetuates the silence surrounding stillborn children. They cite Stanford Bourne's 1977 letter in the *British Medical Journal*, in which he noted that the first British paper on stillbirth (written by him) was published in 1968 in *The Journal of the Royal College of General Practitioners*. In addition he notes that the only other reference to stillbirth at that time was in an article in the *Journal of the American Medical Association* from 1962. Bourne argues that "the syndromes around stillbirth include the feature of extraordinary medical resistance to publishing anything about it" (1157). Yee also notices that most studies done on birth bereavement are published in "psychiatric and medical journals, and books rather than those of obstetrics" (122), which only adds to the silence.

Today, few articles are still being written about stillbirths, even though the Centers for Disease Control and Prevention has found that about twenty-four thousand babies are stillborn in the United States, which is ten times the number of children who die from

SIDS (Sudden Infant Death Syndrome) in the United States every year. Even more troubling is P. Turton et al.'s groundbreaking study about whether a relationship exists between experiencing a stillbirth and experiencing PTSD (post-traumatic stress disorder) symptoms in subsequent pregnancies. Their research shows that women who had experienced a stillbirth were associated with PTSD symptoms in later pregnancies, but the symptoms resolve "naturally by 1 year post-partum (birth of healthy baby)" (556). Their work reiterates that the pain of having a stillborn child does not go away quickly, even if society and others do not wish to speak about it. The authors argue "timely intervention also may reduce the likelihood of the re-emergence of symptoms in subsequent pregnancies" (559). Joan Cooper's research in the United Kingdom on the reactions of couples after a stillbirth has shown how silence affects coping strategies. Six couples (out of seventeen total couples) were surprised by how many "friends and acquaintances had experienced a stillbirth without ever previously alluding to it" (61). As years pass, the silence surrounding stillbirths continues.

LEARNING TO GRIEVE

Parents of stillborn children have no choice but to go through the experience. They are dealt a blow they did not ask for.

> I remember not wanting anyone else to hold Andrew except my husband, myself, the attending Physician, and "B," the maternity nurse who had stayed on long past the end of her shift to be with me through the delivery. I just kept staring at Andrew, hoping he would open his eyes. I didn't want any more people in the room. He felt so fragile to me.

Months later, family members would state they had wanted to see him. They, too, said they felt distanced from the event. My husband and I were lucky that we had the chance to hold Andrew for as long as we did. Emanuel Lewis has likened the immediate period after the birth of stillborn children to a "rugby pass," whereby, the baby is delivered, speedily covered and handed out of the room, away from the family (305).

At the individual level, the grieving mother is left to "mother" without a child. This dilemma is troubling and is not voiced within society. What is expected from these now nonmothers? Does society make them invisible to avoid discussing what mothering with loss looks like? How is mothering done in a nontangible manner? Women are also faced with the notion of loving someone who is dead at delivery. The image of a grieving mother cradling her lifeless, stillborn child is a macabre image from horror movies. There is an underlying notion that the woman is odd and is not functioning in reality as she rocks her stiff child. Yet social science research shows otherwise. Stringham et al. note that several women in their study who held their dead babies benefitted from that experience; some wished that "they had held them longer, kissed them, spent time alone with them, or looked at them more closely" (324).

Later that night, I found myself agitated by an aide who was going to take Andrew to the morgue. I didn't want to let him go, but at that point, I was exhausted. I felt she didn't know him, and I didn't trust her. In the middle of the night, I woke up, realized I was in the hospital, and it took me a minute to remember all that had happened. I realized Andrew was in the hospital somewhere and hit the buzzer to call the night nurse. Sobbing, I asked her to bring him back to me so that I could hold him. She said, "I can't do that, I am sorry, I just can't." I wailed in protest. "I just want him back, I just want him back."

Concomitantly, grieving mothers struggle with guilt and shame surrounding their loss. They walk the streets still looking pregnant a few weeks after delivery; they watch other pregnant women, or women pushing strollers with infants, but they know they have no baby to care for.

I remember stepping out onto the busy Chicago street in the warm spring sun. I realized I would see plenty of strollers; Peg Paregos, Maclarens, Bugaboos, and Baby Joggers. It wasn't the strollers I dreaded as much as neighbours and acquaintances that hadn't heard about Andrew's death.

I looked "postpregnant" with my saggy belly, yet I had no stroller to call my own and certainly no one to put in it. I struggled with the paradox of wanting to tell "his" story, but feeling reticent at the same time to relay it, as people always seemed so uncomfortable hearing about his death. Such reactions made me less likely to want to share any details or feelings. Later, when I had my second son, I would dress him up and stroll with him for miles every afternoon. I told myself at the time it was to get him to nap, and although that is true, I think I subconsciously wanted somehow to show that I, too, had become a "real" mom.

Mothers of stillborn children often wonder what role they had in the loss of their child. Lewis argues that grieving mothers struggle with their own "unconscious feelings of shame and guilt," and notes that their "shame is associated with the sense of having failed as [women]" (304). She feels her own thoughts or actions may have caused the death. Such feelings, again, are not shared with anyone and become even more troubling.

I remember thinking through what I had done in the days before March 15th. I replayed my stubborn determination to put furniture protectors under his crib. I had bought them and bent over to place them gently under each leg. I cringed when I thought maybe I had caused Andrew to die by worrying about the state of the wood floors under his crib. Later, after his autopsy showed no particular findings, my obstetrician had ordered tests for STDs. I was horrified, thinking again I might have been at fault. The tests all came back negative. I continued to blame myself. I should have counted fetal kicks. I should have known.

A second problem for grieving mothers occurs at the family level. How does motherhood get constructed for children we can't see, touch, hold, or feel? Our parenting does not continue in the same physical sphere, yet our hearts tell us differently. Both Stringham et al. and Linda Layne argue that parents attempt to create memories to preserve their child. As Stringham et al. note, "With so little opportunity for memories, families cling to small details that may seem unimportant to others. A glimpse of the baby's face, a tender description by a nurse ('she's beautiful and has lots of dark hair')" (325).

In her article, "Making Memories: Trauma, Choice and Consumer Culture in the Case of Pregnancy Loss," Layne, an anthropologist who has dealt with numerous miscarriages, examines three pregnancy loss support groups. She shows how the attendees often deconstruct and battle the typical conceptualizations of motherhood and parenting as being attached to the notion of physical presence and quantity. Because their children are no longer in the room, they worry about the "corroding effects of time on memory" (123). In addition, they have little to hold on to and thus they treasure the "home pregnancy test dipstick ... baby blankets, caps, hospital ID bracelets, locks of hair, photos, foot and hand prints, and perhaps a toy" (126). I remember wondering if I would remember the shape of Andrew's eyes, the dimple in his chin, and his tiny fingers? Would I remember his thick dark locks and his balled up little fists?

I personally deeply regret that I did not hold on to more clothing or other items of his. I have his foot prints and a little polaroid of him taken by the hospital. In all honesty, I can't bring myself to dig it out of my "Andrew box" in my closet these days, as I'm afraid the polaroid might be completely faded and his image truly gone forever.

A third dilemma for parents of stillborn children is the struggle at the broader social level to find a social community to share feelings and stories with about their lost infant. As Lewis notes, "There is no one to talk about and no-one to talk to about it" (304). How do you get people to validate a person whom they never saw, held, or heard? How do you weave a nonliving child into your experience, when he "didn't exist," according to the world's standards? How do you respond when people ask how many kids you have? Or how do you politely avoid scheduling activities on difficult days, such as his birthday or the anniversary of his funeral? This is the ambiguous space of motherhood. G.C.

Forrest et al.'s findings are similar: "Parents often found that relations with friends and acquaintances were difficult in the first few weeks: friends with young children tended to keep away at first, and then perhaps a month or two later assumed that the parents had recovered" (1478).

The research of Karen Kavanaugh and her colleagues confirm Forrest's findings. They present data showing a similar pattern in which some family and friends isolated bereaved parents and did little in terms of offering social support. Their findings expose detailed accounts of parents who felt abandoned by family members, who did not go to the funeral, stopped calling them, or made comments such as "She's in a better world, she's more happy, she probably knows how this world is" (Kavanaugh 78-9). These authors show how bereaved parents may "feel isolated and misunderstood," which "can have lasting effects" (70).

Moreover, in the West pressure exists not to embrace grief but to "get over it." Many people view stillborn children as never living; thus, many are pressured to move on and forget the trauma. Such a difficult combination makes having a conversation about stillborn children even harder to bear. As Layne notes, "the difficulty of finding empathetic interlocutors is one of the most common themes in narratives of pregnancy loss" (124).

In the case of my son, Andrew, there are a few treasured people in my life that even utter his name. It is those very few family members and close, dear friends who have helped me through. Most people, unfortunately, get the look of "Oh my gosh, she's talking about him, now what do I do next?" Most people smile awkwardly and change the subject, a pattern I used to find troubling and now I find simply sad, as they can't talk about death, especially that of youngsters.

In the cases of families who have lost children, the data suggest they want to be asked about their dead children. They want to talk about their sons and daughters. Ignoring them, as if they do not exist, makes the parents' grief much more isolating and dark. Individuals might start by asking about details of when and where the deaths occurred; what the mother remembers most about her pregnancy; or what she imagines that her child would be like now. Such questions, though seemingly frightening to many, are ones that most mothers would relish being asked and would happily respond to.

CONCLUSIONS

The grief surrounding the loss of children, in my case a stillborn child, is simply overwhelming. Parents are grieving "what should have been." Nicol notes that, "The extent of deterioration in mothers' health after the bereavement is highly comparable to levels for widows" (qtd. in Callan and Murray 249). Additionally, Gary Benfield and his colleagues argue on the basis of the data from their parent-grief scores that maternal grief exceeds paternal grief. Such findings leave mothers completely alone. Even partners and spouses do not experience infant loss in the same way the pregnant mother does, and after the death, they often process their grief in different ways. Clearly, women develop strong emotional attachments to the infants they carry that are different from the father's.

> *Even now, years later, I can still remember the day, time, and moment that Andrew gave his last kick. At the time, I didn't realize how significant it was. I trusted their word and believed that "He was fine." I never even knew stillborn babies existed. No one had ever mentioned them. I had heard of SIDS and yet never read chapter sixteen in . on what to expect when something goes wrong. Why would I read that? Why would I get myself upset? I had continued to live in the nonchalant world of happy pregnancy, not knowing what was around the corner for me, my family, or Andrew.*

We cannot measure pregnancy loss with standard, typical bounded notions of parental input and quantifications. The losses are simply too overwhelming to even fully process or understand. These lives are not measured by typical time or history, but they are no less significant. Motherhood in this fluid conceptualization transcends time and space.

For us parents, stillborn children are about possibility and belief, not about tangibility and physical space. I have realized with time that when you lose a child it is not a failure in motherhood; rather, motherhood is redefined. It is motherhood that doesn't make sense, but you learn to live with your child not being in the room, not being at the party, and not heading off to kindergarten on the big yellow bus. It is rethinking how your motherhood affects your life. Andrew's death forced me to think about who I was as a woman without a baby (given I had no other living children). I was cognizant that I had been the mother to an infant for forty weeks, but now I was not sure if I could retain that title. When I raised the issue with a colleague whose office was across the hall, she noted, "Oh, don't worry, you'll be a mother someday," which confirmed my worst fears that I had lost my motherhood status. Additionally, I knew that externally not having an infant nearby meant I could not hastily revive that status. The liminal space of being a "between" or a "sort of" mother felt alienating and isolating. Interestingly enough, such lack of clarity and vague location actually speak to all reproductive bodies. The experience of stillbirth, I believe, allows us to see that mothering is not solely a physical phenomenon involving only the structural-materialist daily tasks of reproducing human capital for a productive society. Rather, it is the everyday, multilayered negotiations of struggling to figure out who we are as women who happen to have reproductive bodies. The dissonance evolves from how, and why, others interpret my maternal body in particular ways and how I subsequently respond to those social constructions. Such answers are, thankfully, ever evolving and changing—not only as women share their stories in books such as this, but also as pregnancy loss hopefully becomes a normative topic, one not relegated to "special chapters" or addendums of "unusual/special cases" in conception, pregnancy, and birth tales.

The ambiguous space of motherhood, then, is in fact not a bounded entity, marked by limited, physical, reified space, but is elastic in nature and is constructed by our children beyond time and space. We do not make ourselves mothers; rather, our children construct us. We would be radically different without them. I, ironically enough, would not be the person I am today without Andrew. Motherhood cannot be conceptualized as just having a child on the floor eating cheerios. It cannot be construed as just having your child physically present. Motherhood comes in many forms and must be recognized in its variety. Even though our children may not appear as present to others, they are always close by.

ENDNOTES

[1] I should note here that two other categories of mothers are also ambiguous in this regard: women who have given up children for adoption and childless women who are awaiting the arrival of said adopted children. Because the women do not have their children present, they fall into the ambiguous space of motherhood. In both cases, loss is part of the identity framework: when adoptive parents lose the promised child and when a mother gives her child up for adoption.

[2] It is important to note that in society individuals are given "value" on the basis of the length of their lives. Individuals who die when they are older are deemed to have had a "good long life"; thus, we presume to understand their deaths. Similarly, youngsters who die suddenly, or without warning, are rightly seen as tragic losses because their lives, which have inherent value, were cut short. What is interesting is that stillborn children are not deemed as having any value, as their lives were seen as "not lived," and, thus, are not worth acknowledging, according to such a value framework. This notion was recently made more clear to me when a pastor mentioned that on gravestones, the dash between two dates represents a valuable, full, lived life. In the case of stillborn children, there is no such dash and only one date is present. That one date, therefore, holds much value, as it signals a life intermingled with death.

WORKS CITED

Benfield, D. Gary, et al. "Grief Response of Parents to Neonatal Death and Parent Participation in Deciding Care." *Pediatrics*, vol. 62, no. 2, 1978, pp. 171-77.

Bourne, Stanford. "Stillbirth, grief and medical education letter." *British Medical Journal* , vol. 1, 1977, pp. 1157.

Callan, Victor J., and Judith Murray. "The Role of Therapists in Helping Couples Cope with Stillbirth and Newborn Death." *Family Relations,* vol. 38, no. 3, 1989, pp. 248-53.

Centers for Disease Control and Prevention. "Facts about Stillbirth." *Centers for Disease Control and Prevention,* 12 Oct. 2016, www.cdc.gov/ncbddd/stillbirth/facts.html. Accessed 8 Sept. 2017.

Cooper, Joan D. "Parental Reactions to Stillbirth." *British Journal of Social Work,* vol. 10, no.1, 1980, pp. 55-69.

Crittenden, Ann. *Price of Motherhood: Why the Most Important Job in the World Is Still the Least Valued.* Henry Holt, 2001.

Forrest, G. C., et al. "Support after Perinatal Death: A Study of Support and Counseling after Perinatal Bereavement." *British Medical Journal,* vol. 285, no. 6353, 1982, pp.1475-79.

Higgins, G. L. "The Lost Infant: Impact on the Family." *Canadian Family Physician,* vol. 26, 1980, pp.1556-59.

Kavanaugh, Karen, et al. "Social Support following Perinatal Loss." *Journal of Family Nursing,* vol. 10, no. 1, 2004, pp. 70-92.

Layne, Linda L. "Making Memories: Trauma, Choice and Consumer Culture in the Case of Pregnancy Loss." *Consuming Motherhood,* edited by Janelle S. Taylor et al., Rutgers, 2004, pp. 122–38.

Lefebvre, Henri. *The Production of Space.* Blackwell, 1991.

Lewis, Emanuel. "Mourning by the Family after a Stillbirth or Neonatal Death." *Archives of Disease in Childhood,* vol. 54, no. 4, 1979, pp. 303-06.

MISS Foundation Online. "Missing Angels Bill Legislation. State Chart," *MISS Foundation,* www.missingangelsbill.org/index.php?option=com_content&view=article&id=76&Itemid=61. Accessed 9 Sept. 2017.

Stringham, Jean G., et al. "Silent Birth: Mourning a Stillborn Baby." *Social Work,* vol. 27, no. 4, 1982, pp. 322-27.

Turton, P., et al. "Incidence, Correlates and Predictors of Post-traumatic Stress Disorder in Pregnancy after Stillbirth." *British Journal of Psychiatry,* vol. 178, June 2001, pp. 556-60.

Yee, Lam Suk. "The Bereaved Mother of a Stillborn." *Journal of the Hong Kong Medical Association,* vol. 38, no. 3, 1986, pp. 121-23.

6.
Full Circle

The Maternal Ambivalence of
a Motherless Daughter

NATALIE MORNING

I T IS WIDELY ASSUMED that motherhood is an eventual occurrence for women. Nancy Russo asserts that despite social, psychological, and scientific advances, biological sex and sex-typing myths are simultaneously linked to motherhood, and an individual's ability, or willingness, to bear children becomes secondary ("The Motherhood Mandate" 144). As mandated motherhood remains an unspoken, yet dominant viewpoint, those falling outside traditional and gendered maternal roles and desires, become marginalized, and are vulnerable toward self-imposed stigma, and the stigma of others. "Today, mother love has achieved the status of a moral imperative. Our current myth holds that the well-being of ... children depends almost entirely on ... an intense, prolonged, and loving bond between mother and child" (Thurer 334).

This emphasis on intensive mothering models became influential in the late 1980s and early 1990s (Douglas and Michaels 4; Badinter 1). The societal concentration of motherhood dubbed the "new momism" attempts to reconfirm the dated discourse that women's work is best expressed through familial endeavours. This parental inclination is often viewed as a modern feminist decision, as opposed to a potentially oppressive and ingrained social norm. Living in a "culture that praises mothers in rhetoric" (Douglas and Michaels 24) gives credibility to the validity of the selfless mother. In *Our Mother's Daughters*, Judith Arcana stresses the idea of the "martyr mother" and contends this patriarchal interpretation of mothering is the "total internalization of traditional ... roles" (15).

Regardless of the cultural refocusing on intensive mothering models, some feel ambivalence toward motherhood. Maternal ambivalence occurs when an individual is indifferent to having children, and a woman's conception of ambivalence may stem from both personal ideals and sociopolitical climates (Brown 122; Badinter 9). In terms of childrearing, the actual practices of intensive motherhood perpetuate unrealistic stereotypes limiting mothers, and shame those failing to meet a particular standard of motherhood or those reluctant to mother (Douglas and Michaels 26). Such standards produce strenuous environments for women ambivalent to motherhood, and these challenges intensify for women who unintentionally become pregnant. One's ambivalence to raising children may change over time. Nevertheless, when faced with unplanned pregnancy, women must engage with their feelings toward childrearing, as they are required to decide whether they will continue to carry.

At the age of twenty-four, I was faced with an unintentional pregnancy, and I had to decide whether or not to have my child. Initially, it was a simple decision—although I had a strong love of children, I had never envisioned myself as a mother. Deciding to obtain an early-term abortion was, in my mind, the only option. Despite the ensuing shock of the pregnancy, I did not wrestle with this decision. And although I did not struggle with my choice to remain childfree, investigating maternal ambivalence in the face of a pregnancy became a time of great trepidation.

Upon securing an appointment to terminate my pregnancy, I faced a two-week waiting period. During this time, despite feeling confident in my decision to move forward with my abortion, I encouraged myself to explore the reasons behind my ambivalence. My dismay did not stem from being pregnant, but from the idea that a time of joy in the lives of so many women, was something I could easily give up. I thought of my own mother—a single mom by choice, who had me at thirty-eight, and died before my fifth birthday. Although we were not together long, I had countless assurances of her love of motherhood, and her determination to have me. I wondered, constantly, what she had been so sure of.

Pregnancy became an unexpected link between my mother and me. As a motherless daughter, I wondered if losing her so young contributed to the ambivalence I felt toward becoming a mother. Confronting my ambivalence allowed me to fully recognize the stigma enveloping abortion. In this chapter, I explore motherless daughters' negotiations of motherhood and pregnancy, and examine how the contradictory politics of abortion further complicate these women's decision to end a pregnancy. I use my experience as a motherless daughter, who has obtained an abortion, to survey how abortion stigma continues to be perpetuated and how identifying as a motherless daughter can affect pregnancy loss.

MOTHERLESS DAUGHTERS, MATERNAL AMBIVALENCE, AND ABORTION

In her text *Of Woman Born*, Adrienne Rich posits that "the loss ... of the mother to the daughter is the essential female tragedy" (237). Although separation from a loved one is acute, a particular immensity encircles the loss of a mother. This gendered conceptualization of motherhood implies mothers are most capable of nurturing children. The mother becomes a paradigm for womanliness and parenthood itself, which, ultimately, leads her offspring to successfully bear children of their own. Furthermore, this highlights a link between mother and daughter based on assumptive and gendered concepts of motherhood and daughterhood.

Motherless daughters are women who have experienced the loss of their mother before they have reached adulthood (Edelman 9). Although most women will become motherless at some point in their lives, this chapter concentrates on those who came into adulthood as motherless daughters. Considering oneself as a motherless daughter requires a degree of self-identification. Whereas I classify myself a motherless daughter through death, others may regard themselves motherless daughters because of neglect or estrangement, just as easily. This is not to insinuate that those who have lost their mothers cannot form bonds with other parental figures, regardless of biological relation, self-mother, or cooperatively mother themselves with others. Nevertheless, establishing oneself a motherless daughter, by name specifically, conjures thoughts of identifying with an experience outside socially constructed concepts of what it is to be mothered.

Intensive models of motherhood are ideals motherless daughters cannot relate to easily. These women have lived on the opposing end of the mothering spectrum because of the absence they experienced. Having lost their mother, motherless daughters may feel as though this approach to motherhood is not questionable, but a form of advice their mother could not pass down, leaving them with the notion that they are incapable of fulfilling a maternal role. Motherless daughters' vigilant focus on the next generation, and their questioning of their ability to mother, can help shape their ambivalence to mother and their decision to terminate a pregnancy. It is onerous to determine a unanimous reason as to why motherless daughters place such intense focus on their own potential motherhood. For motherless daughters, the act of losing their mothers, perhaps, sets into motion an internal deliberation of the meaning of motherhood and their preparedness for that role, because such an example might have been missing from their upbringing.

Motherless daughters struggle with conceptualizing their own vitality. Regardless of whether they have children, or remain childfree, an added anxiety comes when they contemplate motherhood. Motherless daughters have experienced a lasting trauma altering not only their maturation into womanhood but their own reproduction (Edelman 266). Motherless daughters will naturally bring their experience of motherloss into their relationship with their children. This is not to suggest negative consequences for children of motherless daughters; however, if a mother feels her rearing as motherless was especially difficult, she may worry she is unfit to provide the "correct" mothering tools for her children.

For myself, the insecurities I have felt regarding my motherless daughterhood lay less in my prospective ability to mother, but in shifting outside connotations of my loss. Particularly during my formative school age years, I wished deeply I could remove the look of pity from the eyes of playmates' mothers, as my uncle gathered me from school. Although I thought little about the differences between my family's structure compared to others, it was clear from a very young age that the adults surrounding me believed I was missing a fundamental presence. This presence was not that of a devoted guardian, but of a mother, specifically; as if mandated through biological ties to me and to her sex, she would unquestionably be the most apt to provide me love and care.

Interestingly, the perseverance of motherless daughters in the face of life-altering trauma negates the idea of the compulsory, devoted mother. Conjointly, motherless daughters, unable to experience this kind of mothering, often cannot fulfil the role of the dutiful daughter to the mother, and, thus, may not perceive themselves as fit to complete the natural progression to selfless motherhood. The focus on ideal societal roles for both mother and, presumably, daughter do not account for "the agonizing losses that mothering can entail, and the lack of control over the circumstances of their mothering that many women experience" (DiQuinzio 4). The understanding that devoted motherhood is a choice separates those identifying as motherless daughters from the dominant social view that a biological mother's presence is essential for children.

Notwithstanding alternative lived experiences questioning ideal motherhood, these connotations of motherhood remain dominant and can be seen in many iterations, from political rhetoric championing family values to different facets of popular culture. Thus, through the focus on the mother's presence, motherless daughters' experiences have become marginalized. Culturally ingrained archetypes of motherhood encourage the belief that mothers are essential to childrearing, and, inadvertently, silence alternative narratives. Even though this is a position motherless daughters know all too well, it can be overwhelming for motherless daughters who are ambivalent to motherhood. Motherless daughters occupy a social location where their experience of trauma is marginally understood, and their maternal choices are condemned. For motherless daughters seeking abortion due to ambivalence, the combination of their social location and the stigma of abortion is demanding, regardless of their assurance they are making the correct decision for themselves.

I cannot remember a time when others did not assume I would eventually become a mother. In the face of being a motherless daughter, my proclivity to have children somehow became enmeshed with my mother's death. To right this imbalance, people presumed I would advance into motherhood. Although I played with the idea of pregnancy and motherhood as a young girl and in adolescence, I cannot recall a time when I felt certain about having my own children. This is, emphatically, not an issue I have had trouble expressing in my personal, professional, and academic life. Despite identifying my ambivalence and attempting to discover reasons as to why I am unsure of my own maternal instincts, I do not often believe that my ambivalence, or the ambivalence of others, is taken seriously.

I have been told that when I meet the right person my stance on children will change, that I will entertain the thought of having children more when I have completed my academic endeavours, that my biological clock will begin to tick and children will follow, and that I will be an exemplary mother; to remain childfree, thus, would be a waste. I am fortunate enough to be connected to loving and generous humans. I realize their words are meant to be encouraging—a way of providing me with maternal guidance; however, it is frustrating for concepts of life without children to be removed from such discussions. When I became pregnant, I carried this with me. Although I knew I was making the right decision, I still felt as if I were betraying those around me. Not to mention, being encompassed by a sense of disillusionment, as I did not expect to truly confront my ambivalence until later in life.

In a social environment valuing the will to mother, I felt guilt about both my ambivalence toward, and the nature of, my pregnancy. It was as if, perhaps, my lack of biological, maternal presence signaled to others I was incapable of envisioning my own reproductive potential. Motherless daughters pride themselves on their strength and flourish in settings where they can tap into their autonomy (Edelman 254). In turn, these traditional and limited conceptualizations of motherhood as well as the call to mother, further complicated my understanding of myself as a motherless daughter. The experience of becoming pregnant, unwittingly, depleted the strength I had come to derive from that identity.

ABORTION STIGMA, MATERNAL BEREAVEMENT, AND MATERNAL AMBIVALENCE

Encountering stigma "negatively changes the identity of an individual" (Kumar et al. 626). This happens both within an individual

and through commonly accepted social ideals. Scholars have con-
textualized abortion stigma as a "social phenomenon constructed
and reproduced locally" (Kumar et al. 628) through myriad means.
The legality of abortion varies in different countries around the
world and continues to be a polarizing issue highly present in the
media. Although political rhetoric and personal beliefs can shape
views on abortion, an undertone regarding the expectations of
women contributes to abortion stigma. These expectations are
founded on gender identity formation, which is incorrectly linked
to the potential to biologically have children. Such preoccupa-
tions rarely leave space for individualized narratives or concepts
of motherhood, parenthood, or gender, outside of limiting and
stereotypical social standards.

Seeking an abortion breaks the social construction of women
as nurturers, and this contributes to the socially and self-imposed
stigmatization of these women (Norris et al. S51). Motherless
daughters face a similar stigma, as their mothers could not provide
nurturance for them. Grief cycles are nonlinear, and a momentous
life occurrence can often bring back painful memories (Edelman
61). For motherless daughters, the stigma faced from self and from
others after deciding to terminate a pregnancy can heighten their
stress and anxiety, as well as cause them to confront the loss of
their mothers once again. The maternally ambivalent motherless
daughter's ambivalence will add to this stress, as they never felt
inclined to mother in the first place. Moreover, claiming one's
reproductive power challenges dominant gender roles concerning
women and motherhood. These pressing circumstances make
motherless daughters engage with dynamics of intention—a toil-
some notion, juxtaposed with the little control these daughters
often have over their motherlessness.

Upon becoming aware I was pregnant, I researched the early
stages of pregnancy and early-term abortion. I felt compelled
to learn about the changes occurring in my body, and felt determined to prepare myself for the upcoming procedure. I was
acutely aware of abortion debates, but being Canadian, I had
never known a time when any federal restrictions on abortion
existed. Although seeking an abortion was not something I had
anticipated for myself, I was aware I had access to such a service

and was always firmly prochoice. It was important for me that I gained the perspective of other women who had been through this experience, so I purposefully sought out these women's accounts in the hope to quell my fears about my emotional and physical state after the procedure. I was not, however, equipped for the accounts of pregnancy termination I encountered. It was difficult to locate a personal account of abortion that was unapologetic, and most women spoke of having regrets that lasted years, even if they stated they were ambivalent to motherhood.

I was already in the throes of self-stigma. I felt my best efforts to be proactive about contraception had failed. I felt guilty I was pregnant, and I hated a position many longed to be in. At that juncture, my employment centred around children, whom I loved dearly, but the physical changes happening in my body affected my ability to be as active with them as I was previously. I was physically exhausted and could not eat properly. I was constantly nauseous and perpetually tired. Mentally, I was coming to grips with an unexpected moment in my life. I was panicked about the upcoming procedure, and I was trying to hide my physical state from my employers and family. I felt overwhelmed; nevertheless, I was sure of my decision, and I was looking forward to feeling connected to myself again. This changed drastically, however, after reading other women's abortion narratives. My anxiety increased exponentially, and I found myself crying multiple times a day. I felt isolated in a way that I had never experienced before. I had only told my partner and a few trusted friends, but I began to feel distanced from them and wondered if they secretly judged my decision.

I felt shameful that as a motherless daughter, I missed my mother's presence, but was already detached from what could eventually be my offspring. Reading the experiences of others began to make me doubtful of my recovery after my abortion, and despite knowing that I would not have this child, I began to doubt myself and the validity of occupying a position of ambivalence. A cogent connection was forged here, as I found myself questioning two entities I had never previously had: my mother, and a child, both somewhat intangible to me. Unexpectedly, thoughts about my pregnancy loss became entangled with emotions regarding the loss of my mother, all of which related to defying myths of ideal motherhood. I questioned why the distance I felt from my own maternity was, invariably, increasing the distance I felt from daughterhood as well.

Abortion is infrequently associated with motherhood, despite the sociopolitical focus on family values linking them together (Jones et al. 80). Mothering in a nurturing fashion is recurrently viewed as an instinctive quality, leaving no room for hesitation or questioning. Considering abortion, customarily, implies choice and a profound evaluation of motherhood and all that it encompasses. Seeking an abortion, however, does not signify ambivalence to having children. There are numerous reasons why a woman may decide to terminate a pregnancy, yet citing overall maternal ambivalence is rarely a reason women disclose. Additionally, women who do concede ambivalence played a role in their decision to abort are generally referring to a temporary ambivalence—often based on age, relationship status, the ability to provide a stable environment for their children, satisfaction with their lives, and goal completion (Finer et al. 113).

Although an element of ambivalence may be present in common reasons women give for seeking an abortion, these motives remain rooted in the socially acceptable standard of women as inherently nurturing. Women often emphasize the qualities of their lives they feel are not fit for motherhood to explain their decision to abort. This is not to demean the individualized and personal feelings expressed by women who have received an abortion; it is meant to highlight the language used to articulate their decisions. This language is entrenched in cultural myths of motherhood, which assist in stigmatizing abortion; therefore, it is possible for women pursuing an abortion to reflect this stigma onto themselves, further complicating their experience.

By the date of my appointment, I had worked myself into a palpable frenzy. I was terrified about what lied ahead for my partner and me. From my research, I expected to be mobbed by angry protesters and harshly judged by the health professionals overseeing my abortion. What followed was not nearly as intense. I entered the facility with ease and was treated with respect and dignity. As I entered the clinic, I noticed the diversity of women present. They ranged from teenagers to women entering middle age, and they were accompanied by friends, partners, and family members. I expected a sombre tone, but the waiting room reflected the ambiance of a general practitioner's office. I will never truly know how those women felt at that moment, or how they felt afterward, but I felt as if I were the least stable person present. The clinic radiated an aura of acceptance, but it only served to put me more on edge. I wondered how I—the woman who firmly recognized her maternal ambivalence—could be so unsure of my ability to successfully navigate the aftermath of my abortion.

Encountering the difficult experience of others online caused me to question my own ideals, but I am not resentful those are the stories I found. Those women were brave to share their very private and painful experiences in order to assist others who found themselves unexpectedly pregnant, and had to make a life-altering decision. Regardless of the similarities, or differences, in our experiences of intentional pregnancy loss, the personal narratives I found represent the real experiences of women who have lived through an abortion. Although all women negotiate trauma uniquely, have diverse views on motherhood, and have distinct values and belief systems, I find it difficult to imagine that a climate so entrenched in abortion stigma had no effect on my experience and the experiences I encountered. The self-professed guilt and shame women live with after terminating a pregnancy do not represent an innate experience, but one that occurs because of the social climate in which they reside (Cockrill and Nack 973; Kumar et al.; Hessini and Mitchell 626).

Abortion stigma can have long-lasting negative effects, which manifest themselves in a multitude of ways. After the initial surprise of an unplanned pregnancy, women are likely to experience much higher levels of stress and anxiety. Unsurprisingly, women feel the greatest amount of psychological distress immediately preceding their abortion (Bradshaw and Slade 932), as this is the time when their intent becomes reality. Presently, advancements in women's health and wellness must be made to incorporate the destigmatization of abortion services and improve mental health strategies supporting women.

Women must be given a safe space to share their lived experiences to avoid self-shame stemming from repression, as well as to provide those seeking abortion with accounts not shadowed by myth or misconception. Linking those seeking, or moving forward from, an abortion to a community concerned mental and physical wellbeing, can greatly lessen abortion stigma (Cockrill 8; Norris et al. S52). Kate Cockrill suggests that it is important to ensure these groupings are of an equal power balance, use common language, and compellingly, that their members share common goals and motivations for seeking an abortion (9-10). Encouraging commonalities among abortion support group members, though provocative, certainly speaks to the likeminded support that I argue benefits motherless daughters, because acceptance extends from communities of shared experience.

Lastly, although brief counselling sessions are compulsory before most abortion procedures in Canada, follow-up care is mostly designated to family doctors or walk-in clinics, which are based on physical care, not mental health care. One of my biggest apprehensions about seeking an abortion was the mandatory counselling session. Surprisingly, my session with a counsellor proved to be one of the most fruitful and healing aspects of my experience. Nonetheless, I was not granted access postabortion to the counsellor with whom I had built rapport or with any mental health professional. Thus, follow-up appointments with a counsellor, with whom trust and acceptance have already been established, should be more readily offered in the future. Such services may encourage women to write more personal narratives, gradually reduce abortion stigma.

Generally, severe anxiety decreases directly after an abortion and continues to decrease steadily in the weeks following (Bradshaw and Slade 935). Although acute stress may dissipate, women still sense the stigma of abortion after their procedure is complete. Because of the controversy centring around abortion, many women decide keep their abortion a secret from those they are close to. The need for secrecy, which is generated from a fear of being socially ostracized because of having an abortion, can weigh heavily on women and increase their feelings of isolation (Astbury-Ward et al. 3141; Cockrill and Nack 973). Furthermore, women who were ambivalent to having children often perceive they will receive an increased amount of stigma if they disclose their abortion to others (Cockrill and Nack 980).

Like abortion, maternal ambivalence is not often disclosed because it goes against dominate social conceptions of motherhood and womanhood. Similarly, motherless daughters are also weary to disclose their position, as they are concerned they will be seen as embodying less womanliness (Rich 243; Edelman 275; Russo, "Overview" 12). Feeling in opposition to their social climate, these women become oppressed by a culture not representing their lived experiences. Thus, these women need to have protected spaces where they can disclose their understanding of abortion, without the fear of being stigmatized, as their ability to make their positions known assists in their recovery (Astbury-Ward et al. 3144; Cockrill and Nack 987).

MOVING FORWARD

Although I experienced an inordinate amount of stress and anxiety in the days leading up to my abortion, I felt a decrease in my overall distress after the procedure. I felt decidedly altered, however, in the weeks following the abortion. I began to feel confident in my decision, and grateful to be moving forward with my life. As with any crucial life decision, though, my experience has transformed me. Terminating my pregnancy has left me feeling both confident and insecure. Although it was a trying time in my life, I felt a sense of confidence that I confronted my maternal ambivalence and made an informed decision right for me. Despite confirming by ambivalence to motherhood, I now struggle to do this as openly as I once did. After experiencing overpowering feelings of stigma brought on by my pregnancy and subsequent abortion, I believe I have internalized some shame.

Although I did not grieve the loss of a child, I did grieve a loss of a portion of myself that felt in control, careful, and invincible. Reflecting on this experience, I can see how my identity as a motherless daughter has instilled in me the need to feel in control. Being faced with an unexpected pregnancy set in motion a period of self-realization regarding the pressure motherless daughters place on themselves to reduce stigma about their upbringings.

This stress, coupled with confronting maternal ambivalence and abortion stigma, encouraged feelings of personal failure. At times, when attempting to conceptualize motherhood, I feel as if am I not entitled to an opinion. Not only am I a motherless daughter, but I have chosen to be childless. I am satisfied with this decision, but it does not prohibit me from feeling like an outsider, especially as my friends and siblings begin to have children. I still question whether those who know my story support my decision as fully, now that they have children of their own. I wonder whether my hesitance to extend my lineage will prevent my mother from living on through my potential children and me. Mostly, I question what would be different if she was still with me. Would I feel as ambivalent to motherhood as I do? Would I have made the same reproductive choices? Would I have even disclosed my pregnancy to her?

Although these will remain unanswered questions, my journey of intentional pregnancy loss has taught me a great deal. Despite feeling stigmatized as a maternally ambivalent motherless daughter who has had an abortion, I recognize that these positions do not define me. Although they have altered me, they do not make me less deserving of love, compassion, respect, and understanding. I have also realized the need for the continued support of motherless daughters and women struggling with difficult reproductive decisions, as both groups experience ongoing grief and stigma linked to oppressive, socially constructed views of what motherhood ought to encompass. Maternal ambivalence, abortion, and maternal bereavement are not only associated with absence, but connected to motherhood, and this recognition can assist in reducing the stigma of existing in these social locations.

WORKS CITED

Arcana, Judith. *Our Mothers' Daughters*. Shameless Hussy Press, 1979.

Astbury-Ward, Edna, et al. "Stigma, Abortion, and Disclosure—Findings from a Qualitative Study." *The Journal of Sexual Medicine*, vol. 9, no. 12, 2012, pp. 3137-147.

Badinter, Elizabeth. *The Conflict: How Modern Motherhood Undermines the Status of Women*. Metropolitan Books, 2011.

Bradshaw, Zoë, and Pauline Slade. "The Effects of Induced Abortion on Emotional Experiences and Relationships: A Critical Review of the Literature." *Clinical Psychology Review*, vol. 23, no. 7, 2004, pp. 929-58.

Brown, Ivana. "Ambivalence of the Motherhood Experience." *21st Century Motherhood*, edited by Andrea O'Reilly, Columbia University Press, 2010, pp. 121-39.

Cockrill, Kate, and Adina Nack. "'I'm Not That Type of Person': Managing the Stigma of Having an Abortion." *Deviant Behavior*, vol. 34, no. 12, 2013, pp. 973-90.

Cockrill, Kate Crosby. "Contact Theory—And How We Can Use it to Destigmatize Abortion." *Ansirh Blog*, 23 July, 2012, blog. ansirh.org/2012/07/contact-theory-and-destigmatizing-abortion/. Accessed 14 Sept. 2017.

DiQuinzio, Patrice. *The Impossibility of Motherhood: Feminism, Individualism, and the Problem of Mothering*. Routledge, 1999.

Douglas, Susan J., and Meredith W. Michaels. *The Mommy Myth: The Idealization of Motherhood and How it Has Undermined Women*. Simon and Schuster, 2004.

Edelman, Hope. *Motherless Daughters: The Legacy of Loss*. Dell Publishing, 1994.

Finer, Lawrence B., et al. "Reasons US Women Have Abortions: Quantitative and Qualitative Perspectives." *Perspectives on Sexual and Reproductive Health*, vol. 37, no. 3, 2005, pp. 110-18.

Jones, Rachel K., et al. "'I Would Want to Give My Child, Like, Everything in the World': How Issues of Motherhood Influence Women Who Have Abortions." *Journal of Family Issues*, vol. 29, 2008, pp. 79-99.

Kumar, Anuradha, et al. "Conceptualizing Abortion Stigma." *Culture, Health & Sexuality*, vol. 11, no. 6, 2009, pp. 625-39.

Norris, Alison, et al. "Abortion Stigma: A Reconceptualization of Constituents, Causes, and Consequences." *Women's Health Issues*, vol. 21, no. 3, 2011, pp. S49-S54.

Rich, Adrienne. *Of Woman Born*. W.W. Norton and Company Inc., 1976.

Russo, Nancy Felipe. "The Motherhood Mandate." *Journal of Social Issues*, vol. 32, no. 3, 1976, pp. 143-52.

Russo, Nancy Felipe. "Overview: Sex Roles, Fertility and the

Motherhood Mandate." *Psychology of Women Quarterly,* vol. 4, no. 1, 1979, pp. 7-15.

Thurer, Shari L. "The Myths of Motherhood: How Culture Reinvents the Good Mother." *Maternal Theory: Essential Readings,* edited by Andrea O'Reilly, Demeter Press, 2007, pp. 331-344.

III. REFRAMING PREGNANCY LOSS

7.
Reframing the Devastation and Exclusion Associated with Pregnancy Loss

A Normal and Growth-Enhancing Component of the Physiological Female Continuum

KEREN EPSTEIN-GILBOA

E VENTS ASSOCIATED with the female physiological continuum, such as birth, are described as transformative experiences (Epstein-Gilboa, *Systems Interaction*; *Interaction and Relationships*, "Maternal Ambivalence"; Rabuzzi; Slade et al.; Stern and Bruschweiler-Stern). Pregnancy loss is a component of some women's continuum often portrayed as a negative experience associated with grief (Davis; Lok and Neugebauer; Madden; Paloma-Castro et al.). The interpretation of loss and depth of mourning is individual and does not seem contingent upon the cause or length of the pregnancy (Klier et al.; Madden; Robinson; Wright and Perry). Miscarriage and birth loss may be complicated by self-blame, guilt, shame (Borg and Lasker; Davis; Madden; Robinson; Wright and Perry), and a sense of failure and damage (Hsu et al.), which may contribute to lingering depression or anxiety (Brier; Geller et al.; Lok and Neugebauer; Robinson). The loss of a pregnancy may also be perceived as traumatic (Lee and Slade) and put women at risk for post-traumatic stress disorder (PTSD) (Robinson). These descriptions seem to suggest that pregnancy loss is a deviation from normalcy impairing emotional growth. However, it appears processes associated with perinatal loss may enhance development for some women (Wright and Perry). This chapter explores the emotionality of pregnancy loss by looking at obstacles impeding healthy emotional growth and by discussing possible means of reframing negativity into a positive transformative experience.

The difficult emotions associated with pregnancy loss—including guilt, a sense of failure, and shame—concur with "disenfranchised grief" (Doka). This concept provides insight into possible barriers to emotional wellbeing following loss. Disenfranchised grief implies one's reasons for mourning and loss are disregarded by others. The mourner perceives their bereavement is unworthy and hides their feelings. Evidence suggests disenfranchised grief may be a reality for women silenced and isolated by culturally condoned taboos devaluing the emotionality of pregnancy loss. Consequently, women fail to seek badly needed support (Austin-Smith; Malacrida; Martel: Mulvihill and Walsh; Robinson; Rowlands, and Lee; Wojnar et al.). Joyce Solomon has described the emotional turmoil she suffered because of religious regulations prohibiting her from mourning an infant less than thirty days of age. Her case exemplifies a means of shutting out women, and the consequences of disregarding their experiences. Thus, the concept of disenfranchised grief shows how distraught women may internalize the idea that a lost pregnancy is not worth grieving and they should forget and get on with life.

Models of psychotherapy help to understand the detrimental effect of silencing women following a loss. Accordingly, openly sharing feelings with empathetic people facilitates emotional wellbeing (Rogers). Moreover, research on trauma emphasizes that the failure to process traumatic events, such as pregnancy loss, may put one at risk for multiple psychological problems, including anxiety, depression, and PTSD (Van der Kolk). With PTSD, traumatic events remain unresolved, and unrelated events may trigger sensations associated with the original trauma. PTSD can be resolved through psychotherapeutic models allowing one to acknowledge and work through feelings associated with the perceived traumatic event (Van der Kolk; Levine; Shapiro).

Helping women change beliefs prolonging pain, such as thoughts associated with guilt and shame, can also promote emotional growth. Cognitive behavioural methods may help women change denigrating thoughts into more helpful ones (Ellis). Mindfulness may contribute to enriched self-awareness, acceptance, and wellbeing by helping one notice thoughts, feelings, and sensations in the present tense without judgment (Kabat-Zinn). Noticing thoughts as separate entities can help one accept associated feelings and at the same time enhance one's ability to integrate more functional beliefs and behaviours (Hayes et al.). One may also help women feel differently about their experience by helping them change the way that they tell their story (White). For example, a woman devastated by perceived humiliation during pregnancy loss will change her position in her story from one of helplessness into one in which she becomes the central and empowered character.

The brief review of literature indicates that women sometimes perceive pregnancy loss as a devastating experience impeding emotional growth. Pain may be exacerbated by pressure to deny and refrain from mourning. Consequently, women may feel silenced, disempowered, deficient, and isolated when they are denied feelings associated with a normal human experience. Moreover, all of these negative feelings distance women from sensing their experience as part of the transformative female continuum. Psychotherapeutic models show how providing women with support and a means of exploration can alter this sad reality and promote emotional wellbeing by. In the next sections, I refer to personal and professional insights as well as established psychological models to demonstrate a means of reframing pregnancy loss as a normal developmental event that may facilitate growth.

MY STORY

For over three decades, I have been supporting women and their families as they experience the physiological continuum of pregnancy, birth, breastfeeding, and mothering. It was my conviction that this continuum influences female development and facilitates a sense of wellbeing, self-actualization, agency, and normalcy. I still believe that these factors significantly affect female development. However, my experience of pregnancy loss has added a new dimension to my thinking. Since early childhood, I have listened to my mother's narrative of birth and mothering reinforcing the cultural idealization of these events. I internalized views about the importance of natural processes while absorbing my mother's proud tale of how she managed to overcome my breech presentation and medical pressure and to birth me naturally. My reverence for women's capacity to experience the natural female continuum was fortified during my training as a nurse in a program that included basic midwifery and provided abundant support for mothers and infants. I perceived that I was on the path to actualizing my lifelong goal when I gave birth naturally and breastfed my daughter for several years. I adored all aspects of the pregnancy, birth, breastfeeding, and mothering continuum so much that I became a childbirth educator, a La Leche League Leader volunteer breastfeeding counsellor, and a lactation consultant long before it was in style. I continued this speciality during my graduate studies in psychology: researching, writing about, and also working with women experiencing the pregnancy, birth, breastfeeding and early parenting continuum in various capacities. I became involved and active in the clinical and political world of physiological pregnancy, birth, breastfeeding, and mothering. Thus, I was devastated when my membership in the community of women experiencing what I perceived as the healthy physiological continuum that I supported was threatened by unexpected miscarriage and loss.

My series of miscarriages took place as I attempted to bring a second child into this world. I had withheld having another child because of my anxiety associated with my firstborn's congenital condition. Physicians told me that my newborn daughter was severely visually impaired only a short time after I had given birth for the first time. The strength I gained through natural birthing and breastfeeding helped me mother this wonderful child. Her function far surpassed the medical prognosis. However, I retained the shock and fear of possibly birthing a child with a worse condition. I was finally ready to have another child only many years after my first daughter was born. I looked forward to re-experiencing a woman-focused and natural style of pregnancy and birth. I wanted to experience the kind of birth I had supported for others, and had taught, wrote, and researched about. My plans were to have a midwife-supported home birth, breastfeed again for years, and engage in an attachment-focused mothering style.

I perceived my first miscarriage at seven weeks as normal and acceptable. I became more anxious after nearly dying from sepsis following the next miscarriage at thirteen weeks. The roles and boundaries of newly government sanctioned and funded midwifery was unclear at the time, in 1994. Thus, despite hiring midwives, I erroneously called on physicians when I suddenly became ill. The physicians missed the urgency of my condition and let me linger in a life-threatening situation. A midwife on call, whom I never met, saved my life by listening to me carefully on the phone and directing me to go the hospital immediately. The hospital protocols at in the early 1990s did not include ongoing midwifery care in the emergency room. I was forced to cope with the eventual diagnosis of sepsis and almost dying, as well as with a dead fetus, and discomfort, all without adequate support. The experience of isolation, fear, confusion, humiliation, and anxiety challenged my former sense of self and long held beliefs.

Anxiety following my second miscarriage clouded future decision making. I decided to work with physicians for the first part of the next pregnancy, and hoped to switch to midwives in the second trimester. I discussed my plans with the midwife with whom I had hoped to work with later on in the pregnancy. Unfortunately, she supported my decision to work with physicians without discussing alternative plans. I believe now she should have been truthful about the implications of medical services, especially for women with my philosophy. Instead, she should have supported me to make use midwifery care instead of agreeing so easily with my decision to use physicians. In my view, she was likely trying to be respectful and offer me choice. However, "choice," a concept originally intended to advance respect, has instead been misconstrued and used without discretion in Western healthcare. Consequently, some service providers may use the word choice in order to seem supportive when in reality they may not actually be committed to advancing the client's status or true intents. In some cases the word choice serves as a means of appeasing, silencing, controlling and isolating rather than advocating for clients (Epstein-Gilboa, "Breastfeeding"). From my perspective at the time, the midwife's immediate acceptance of my decision to use the services of medical physicians for part of my pregnancy rather than trying to convince me to use midwifery implied that I was different, deficient, and unworthy of midwifery support. I could no longer trust my own physiology and required medical care. Choice in this case actually left me isolated and feeling there was no other option other than to turn to physicians.

The physicians were condescending. They disputed my views of natural processes and constantly reminded me I had miscarried previously. They said that I was at risk and my body could not grow a baby on its own. I was told to trust their patriarchal processes that included but were not limited their constant use of technology, their belief pregnancy was dangerous and their view of themselves as saviours. These medical professionals repeatedly told me that I was to stop thinking like a nurse and a woman with experience. They used the term "patient" instead of "client." They stated clearly that I was to act like a patient and let them make the decisions for me.

I managed to retain some of my belief in physiology, albeit with a reduced sense of agency, until I noticed a small amount of bleeding. At that point, I lost my good judgment and allowed the physician to interfere and remove a polyp. This procedure like other aggressive interventions associated with the medical model put my pregnant body at risk for infection and complications. During pregnancy, mothers are more susceptible than the general population and may have severe responses to certain pathogens (Mor and Cardenas). The inflammatory response may lead to negative consequences including preterm birth and developmental abnormalities (Racicot et al.). My experience working with midwives using a women-centred model respectful of physiology and minimal intervention suggests they would not have put my body at risk the way that the physicians did. Less than two weeks after the erroneous removal of the polyp, I began experiencing uterine contractions. The contractions were so intense that I used Lamaze coping skills I had taught for years and had helped me birth naturally years earlier. My capacity to cope with labour pains without intervention was beyond the medical team's scope of understanding. They denied the gravity of the situation and my perception of recurring pain as contractions. I repeatedly tried to explain to the physicians about physiology and women's capacity to birth without their medication. They belittled my conviction I was in labour and needed help. One pompous specialist ridiculed me: "women [in their second pregnancies] have pain and you are going to have more." Ten days later, I stopped believing in myself, apologized for being a nuisance, and ceased complaining. After two weeks of suffering contractions and pain far exceeding my previous birthing experience, I gave birth to my nineteen-week-old live son while I was alone at home with my daughter. I will never forget the horror I felt when I realized that I was birthing my baby. I still see him moving frantically in my arms and can still taste his salty skin. My then twelve-year-old daughter called the emergency services while I applied CPR, trying unsuccessfully to save my son's life. We lost the battle, he died, and I felt I had lost part of myself.

The medical team continued their quest of enforcing their apparent superiority through messages about pathology, risk, weakness, and my vulnerability after my son's death. Scare tactics succeeded at pressuring me to agree to a dilation and curettage (D&C) when the placenta refused to separate. This medical intervention, similar to the one that had caused the premature birth, damaged my body. The ligaments in my legs were destroyed forever. Later, it became apparent that I was also rendered infertile. I was deemed "high risk" for future pregnancies. The physicians commanded that I comply with medical procedures I find repugnant. I was told firmly I was to refrain from using the services of woman-focused midwives should I ever become pregnant again. This was horrifying for me considering my personal and professional investment in women-centred physiology and services. I now felt like a failure and physiologically deficient. Unfortunately, the midwife I contacted earlier reinforced my sense of exclusion. Without meaning to, she conveyed that I was no longer "midwife worthy" when she failed to contact me other than to give me blood reports a few weeks after the loss and only after I had left her several messages. However, the physicians were the focus of my distress and anger. I reported the medical specialist who had ignored and belittled my capacity to assess my condition to his professional college. I sank deeper into depression after I lost the case, and my appeal was denied despite my well-researched presentation. Thus, interactions with health service providers were a source of pain and contributed to the devastation and exclusion I felt at all levels.

The relentless pain and grief associated with pregnancy loss is greater than any other bereavement I have ever experienced. In fact, I write this chapter while mourning the loss of my most beloved mother. The ambivalence and guilt associated with losing a parent feels less intense than with a lost pregnancy. My grief for my mother is open and supported. Even though it is painful, people expect to lose their parents. However, I never expected to lose an infant. Furthermore, all of my miscarriages were complicated by trauma exceeding that of losing a parent. In the case of my last pregnancy, I had to cope with extreme and unrecognized physical pain as well as the shock of birthing a live infant whom I attempted to save. These memories were accompanied by guilt and initial shame and prevented me from receiving the same support as I had following the death of my mother. While grieving my mother, I can refer to happy memories for support. In place of actual positive memories of my mother, I mourn fantasies of what the child might have been like. I have watched my child grow in my head for the past twenty-two years knowing I will never be able to talk with, watch, or hold him. Grief is fortified further by sadness for my daughter who never had siblings and from knowing our family is incomplete. One also loses cherished functions. I lost my longed-for physiological pregnancy and home birth at term with supportive midwives and future fertility. This type of loss leaves one feeling barren, disappointed, alone, deficient, different, and cheated. I found bereavement following pregnancy loss to be most difficult because of my perception it deviated from a normal expected life course and also because of the complexity of associated feelings.

I attempted to cope with my feelings of deficiency, hopeless-ness, extreme sadness, self-blame, and guilt by speaking to a kind psychotherapist who had also lost her own babies. However, I never felt worthy enough to join a badly needed pregnancy loss bereavement group. I thought most mothers in the group would have lost full-term infants. I felt less worthy than those mothers considering I had not carried my baby to term. I also felt selfish and uncomfortable talking about my loss beside women who did not have other children when I was fortunate enough to have one child. In addition, I felt deficient in comparison to mothers who could successfully birth or raise more than one child. I felt different from most women and could not speak in most circles.

My professional obligations increased the severity of my tor-turous trajectory to healing. Feelings of distress were exacerbated as I fulfilled the role as lactation consultant on a maternity unit only two weeks after burying my son. The constant reminder of my inability to fulfill tasks I did for others reinforced my sense of loss and exclusion. On one hand, I was open and told others I had recently lost a baby son. On the other hand, I conformed to silencing by denying the gravity of my pain. During this time, I also engaged in unsuccessful fertility treatments causing me undue pain, not only because of my failure to conceive, but also because of interactions with insensitive practitioners I met along the way. I tried to distance myself from my own experience as I advocated for women and helped them nurse babies the same gestational age as my son who lay in a cold grave.

Strangely enough, work with mothers began to draw me closer to healing insights. I visited mothers who had lost babies on the maternity unit, even though this was not part of my role as lactation consultant. I wanted to convey a sense of camaraderie, mutuality, normalcy, and acceptance that had been withheld from me. I also began to help women in my private practice and personal life who had endured loss. I discovered the women I met shared many of my feelings. I noted how my own experience provided me with new tools to speak and help other women. I began to create novel scripts about pregnancy loss I had never thought of previously.

THE CREATION OF NOVEL SCRIPTS OF PREGNANCY LOSS

Although I continued to experience loss and anger, I also began to see my miscarriages as treasured rather than deviant events. I realized I was privy to valuable insights that I never would have had without my loss. This new knowledge was exciting. Most importantly, my own experience allowed me to feel more comfortable working with women after their loss. Disclosing that I had also lost a baby encouraged them to share their stories with me. Similar to my decision to see a psychotherapist who had experienced loss, these women disclosed feelings to me they withheld from other nurses or therapists who did not belong to this group. I not only enjoyed my ability to help women in a way I could not before, but I also cherished the newfound insights that came to light about this formerly hidden experience of womanhood.

The physiological continuum was my term of reference for normalcy prior to experiencing loss and iatrogenic (caused by medical intervention) secondary infertility. I turned to this same continuum but with a different perspective. I became increasingly cognizant of the salience of loss for the female continuum. I realized the revered female continuum also included the loss of unfertilized ovum, embryos, fetuses, and infants. These essential events have occurred from the start of time. I also noted the similarity between silencing following miscarriage and the act of hiding other female losses. For example, for most of my life, the simple but prevalent act of losing an unfertilized ovum (i.e., menstruation) was also only spoken about in whispers.

So here I was now privy to a silenced component of women's life cycle. My membership provided me entry into a new world. I celebrated these new insights about female experiences with physiological and historical significance. I increasingly acknowledged the positive impact my devastating loss had on my way of understanding the world; it elevated me as a person and advanced my clinical skills. I began to formulate novel scripts based on my newfound ways of knowing, and I began to reframe pregnancy loss. In the next section, I refer to the insights gained through my personal experience as well as observations of and discussions with peers and clients who had experienced pregnancy loss.

SHARED THEMES

My observations and analysis of women's patterns and themes were comparable to aspects of my personal experience and the existing literature. The wide array of emotional expressions experienced by these women included the following: feelings associated with trauma, sense of failure, regret, guilt, self-blame, shame, envy, anger, hopelessness, anxiety, longing for the lost child and future, discomfort with emotional sharing, and a sense of isolation and exclusion. In my experience, many women were overwhelmed by intense emotional pain immediately following the loss. Pain intensity and the type of emotion changed over time for many women. For example, in some cases, a feeling of self-blame changed to one of longing as time passed. However, resolved negativity could be triggered at any time. Most women retained complex but varied emotional residue regardless of the stage of pregnancy, type of pregnancy loss, the childbearing experience, or amount of time following the loss.

I noted individuality and diversity in women's narratives. Some spoke about past miscarriages and related pain as if they endured the loss in the present tense. This finding suggests that some might have been suffering from post-traumatic stress. Others recounted their tales in a distant style. Moreover, the same person might have different reactions to pregnancy loss depending on related life experiences. For example, a woman who endured years of infertility and recurrent miscarriages found it more difficult to cope with miscarriages after giving birth to a healthy child. For her, miscarriage was most difficult after becoming a mother because she knew what she was missing. For other women, their emotional pain was more severe before they had given birth to live children. Their grief was complicated by a sense of emptiness and anxiety about childlessness. Individuality is an obvious factor when considering the impact of pregnancy loss on women's development.

Although women's stories were unique, they also shared some elements. The sense of being silenced, excluded, and negative self-regard were prevalent themes, and they influenced one another. Themes were sustained by women's views of themselves in relation to pregnancy loss as well as their interactions with others.

Negative self-regard interfered with the women's ability to discuss bereavement and to feel included in relevant social circles. The terms many women used to refer to themselves in relation to pregnancy loss demonstrated shame and self-loathing. These included failure, leper, pariah, deviant, and worthless.

Self-blame, guilt, shame, and regret were particularly encompassing and distressful in the early period following miscarriage. The severity of associated emotions seemed to decrease significantly over time. However, these themes continued to appear periodically and to influence women's self-regard in later narratives.

Women's perceptions of their worthiness were multilayered and included long-standing personal viewpoints. Some attached self-worth to the quality of their physiological processes. In this case, one's perceived inability to actualize revered physiological tasks was a source of self-imposed devaluation. Women growing up in families or cultures associating health, normalcy, and worth with the capacity to reproduce may link the loss of a physiological function with a negative view of self. These narratives also triggered a sense of worthlessness when one could not fulfil self-generated goals. Thus, culture, family, and individual meaning contributed to a sense of devaluation based on one's perceived inability to actualize cherished functions.

Women's perceptions of their experiences compared to those of other women also influenced their self-regard. I repeatedly heard women state how they felt inferior to women who could actualize fertility-related tasks that they could not. Women compared themselves to counterparts with successful reproductive experiences as well as those with relatively longer pregnancies than they had experienced prior to miscarrying. Comparisons with other women led some to feel they were not as successful or could not achieve what other women could. The desire to be liked or to have an unattainable object owned by another is associated with envy (Klein). In this case, the envied object was functional reproductive capacities. Envy might have contributed to some women's sense of exclusion and reduced their ability to speak about their pain. Women's perceptions of relative suffering also played a role in their self-esteem and capacity to share feelings. Accordingly, some women implied that they felt less valuable and their right to mourn was invalid compared to women who, apparently, had endured more devastation. Thus, the reasons why some women felt less credible than others varied. However, in all cases, a reduced sense of self further contributed to feelings of devaluation and silencing as well as to creating a distance between sisters who could have provided badly needed support to one another.

Women's disgust with others was another central theme. Messages perceived by women as derogatory contributed to feelings of worthlessness, silencing, and exclusion. Some women exhibited rage, frustration, and an increased sense of insignificance when they felt others either forgot or minimized their pregnancies. They felt devalued when their trauma and lost babies were ignored. Some recounted the distress they felt when they were apparently blamed or told not to talk about their loss. It was difficult to ascertain the true intent of others in women's narratives. Some perceptions might have reflected other's actual words or viewpoint. In some cases, the cruelty might have mirrored women's attributions about others' intentions and their own inner voices. Either way, women's perceptions of culturally condoned messages and taboos regarding pregnancy loss contributed to negative self-regard, silencing, and feelings of exclusion.

My personal experience, observations, and analysis of themes concur with existing findings about the complex emotional trajectory following pregnancy loss as well as the centrality of devaluation, silencing, isolation, and exclusion in women's scripts. For some women, the loss of a pregnancy, infant, and fertility implies they have also lost an important part of what they had hoped to be and to accomplish. Pregnancy loss also represents lost membership and community. I use these insights as I support women and help them facilitate a process of reframing devastation into growth.

INTERVENTION: LISTEN, VALIDATE, NORMALIZE, ACCEPT, AND RETELL THE STORY

The concept of positive transformation following painful female experiences is increasingly noted in the current literature on miscarriage aftermath (Wright) and postpartum depression (Karraa). In my work, I support growth by using set psychotherapeutic concepts. I also rely on my personal insights and attempt to be sensitive to each woman's unique cues and state of readiness. The psychotherapeutic tools I use may include empathy, validation, anticipatory guidance, and reframing. I sometimes provide a means of processing traumatic events and help women alter thoughts stifling growth. Some clients may feel relief through mindfulness and by accepting their process. When appropriate, I refer to feminist concepts and the influence of culture on women's views of self. I help women reconstruct their stories in a manner encouraging positive self-regard and emotional growth. I always bear in mind the reality of coping with grief in cultures that belittle pregnancy loss and deprive women of their right to mourn.

The first step required in reconstructing a story is to help women overcome the experience of silencing and avoidance. One may counter these experiences by demonstrating respect and showing a woman that one is genuinely interested in listening to her story. Validating and accepting a woman's emotions are essential tools in this process (Rogers). In my case, I am "lucky" and may break the ice by disclosing portions of my own experience. This action reduces isolation and enhances feelings of normalcy. However, it is important to remember the salience of exclusion even within the group of women sharing miscarriage history. Thus, a therapist must initially withhold parts of her story that might be portrayed as more credible than the other woman's experience. The therapist should add portions of her story to suit the level of readiness to the grieving mother's cues.

Listening, validating, and demonstrating genuine positive regard (Rogers) implies refraining not only from judging the other woman, but also from trying to make her feel better. Efforts to remedy another woman's horrid experiences without her initiative or engagement can mimic cultural silencing. Instead, one should help a woman know feelings such as envy and guilt are normal. These feelings can promote growth when one is able to psychologically repair perceived damage (Klein). An important component of the reframing process is to show acceptance and openness about apparently deviant feelings. The sense of being heard is an important healing step leading one to form healthier ideation.

Some women are too overwhelmed by trauma to discuss their feelings and to receive the optimal validation. This again may be the result of silencing that forces them to hide details of the traumatic loss. Thus, some women try to bury their trauma. Buried experiences, however, remain very much alive in one's memory causing one to intermittently feel sensations, such as fear for example, directly associated with the trauma. We might correct the experience of silencing by helping women confront, revisit, and process concealed memories (Bessel; Levine; Shapiro). The goal of trauma work is to allow a woman to remember while she feels safe and distant from the frightening sensations associated directly with the traumatic loss. Dealing with trauma may resolve all of the pain for some. For other women, processing is only an initial step allowing them to continue challenging their perspective of pregnancy loss and sense of exclusion.

Cognitive behavioural techniques can challenge apparently irrational beliefs and change obstructive thoughts into functional thinking (Ellis). I say this with caution and realize the definition of functional thoughts is individual. One should take into account the unique features of pregnancy loss. For example, self-blaming seems to be inherent to many women's processes and contributes to a sense of exclusion. On one hand, the therapist may challenge conceptualizations reinforcing self-blame by exploring the source, interpretation, and rationality of intrusive thoughts. On the other hand, the counsellor might respect the women's rate of change and merely provide anticipatory guidance about the role of self-blame in the grieving process. Some women feel a sense of relief when they learn their feelings and thoughts are shared by others under similar conditions. Notions of mutuality normalize apparently deviant emotions and increase a sense of inclusion.

Realistic information helps women set healthy goals and reduce self-denigration. Unfortunately, some women are challenged by external sources of faulty thinking. For example, they internalize negative thoughts associated with medically aligned literature indicating deviance from a set pattern of mourning after pregnancy loss is pathological (Lok and Neugebauer). One woman's interactions with a physician following an earlier pregnancy loss exemplify the potentially harmful effects of misguided thinking. This woman revealed she was still mourning her stillborn infant to the physician attending the subsequent pregnancy two years after the loss. The physician was apparently appalled she was still mourning her lost infant and immediately prescribed antidepressant medication rather than validating her process. Needless to say, the physician's message increased this woman's concerns about her current pregnancy and ability to mother her expected baby. This mother's story, as well as others, indicates many women continue to experience painful feelings about past miscarriages that may be periodically triggered regardless of the length of pregnancy or quality of miscarriage. In my experience, anticipatory guidance about realistic information—such as individualized mourning periods and the knowledge that negatives feelings may reoccur after apparent resolutions—may paradoxically reduce re-occurrence.

Guidance normalizing an individual's experience can reduce stress and advance feelings of inclusion. I sometimes combine knowledge and anticipatory guidance with methods helping women see their emotions as separate entities (Ellis; Hayes et al.). Thoughts are seen as transient independent objects to be noticed rather than as powerful and controlling internal states. These tools allow women to become aware of feelings while helping their negative emotions dissipate. In other words, I help women who seem overwhelmed by their sense of sadness to accept their emotions without ruminating about the reasons for the negativity or how they might feel in the future. The thought is accepted without a need for change. Accepting feelings also advance women's ability to commit to more functional scripts promoting wellbeing (Hayes et al.). These tools can reduce anxiety in the present and during instances when uncomfortable feelings resurface. Through these techniques, women learn they need not rid themselves of negative emotions; they may accept the pain and the right to never forget. Acceptance may decrease exhaustion associated with fighting apparent negativity. Acknowledging, allowing, and accepting the process is congruent with positive self-regard and feelings of inclusion.

Concepts associated with feminist therapy (Jordan) suggest that growth may be facilitated by providing information and discussing women's perception of the impact of systemic messages on self as woman and in relation to pregnancy loss. Insights about unresolved patriarchal envy of female capacity imply that males envy, belittle, and show contempt toward and try to destroy those fortunate enough to experience those events (Epstein-Gilboa, *Systemic Interaction*; *Interaction and Relationships*; "Breastfeeding"). Thus, negative notions of miscarriage can serve an important function for patriarchal bodies. The preservation of miscarriage as negative and as a sign of deficiency enables patriarchal sources to silence and triumph over strong women. My experiences and those of other women indicate some of our negative self-perceptions may stem from interchanges with patriarchal medical systems invested in preserving female weakness. For example, I frequently disclose the example of a physician (nicknamed as "the cowboy" by nurses behind his back) who subtly implied that I was weak and vulnerable by trying to hide pregnant women from me during an ill-fated appointment after I lost my baby. His apparent attempts to protect me were not only inappropriate but also belittling considering he knew I worked daily with pregnant women, mothers, and babies. He eventually refused to provide me services under the pretence that I failed to trust him fully and my apparent mistrust of his skills could endanger me. In reality, I believe he was threatened by my strength and ability to cope with pregnancy loss. He felt uncomfortable with his perceived inability to actualize protection and his need to heal what he saw as a physiologically defective woman.

Distancing from patriarchal influence and internalizing a sense of agency is further developed by referring to women's unique wisdom and connection to physiology (Northrup). In my clinical practice, I discuss my novel conceptualization of the female continuum when a client shows signs of readiness to integrate new concepts into her system. We talk about redefining the culturally set perspective of women's physiological continuums to include miscarriage, infant death, and loss as central to women's stories and lives. Instead of viewing loss as an outlier, we redefine associated experiences as central components of the female physiological continuum. We look at history and refer to historically revered female characters who experienced pregnancy loss. We frame pregnancy loss as a significant and uniquely female experience. This experience provides one with a true sense of the female trajectory, inclusive of unique insights and windows to the world and strength.

Additional insights into women's way of knowing, inclusion, and agency may be facilitated by reconnecting to valued parts of the self pre-trauma (Herman). Women acknowledge that former cognitive, behavioural and physiological parts of the self do continue despite apparent reproductive failure. At times, I may guide women by asking questions that help them refer to things they liked about themselves prior to and during the pregnancy, miscarriage, or aftermath. Reconnecting to the healthy self acknowledges existing function in a seemingly dysfunctional body. This viewpoint counters the message of overall dysfunction that was evident in some women's experiences with medical systems. In contrast, my position is that multiple parts of the physical and psychological self may work exceedingly well despite the difficulties in one area. In this case, one may help women acknowledge and celebrate functional parts of their physiology. Women's use of breastfeeding as compensation for perceived physiological failure demonstrates how women may use one physiological experience to help resolve the perceived loss of another component of their trajectory. Findings indicate, for example, that mothers who have not carried and birthed biological children may view their breast-feeding relationships with adopted children as compensation for lost functions (Epstein-Gilboa, *Systemic Interaction*; *Interaction and Relationships*). This paradigm can also alter the meaning of distressing components of miscarriage. For example, in certain cases, I have reframed the disturbing connotations of breast engorgement following stillbirth into signs of health, normalcy, a working body, and hope for the future. Helping a woman see that she can still trust parts of her physiology compensates for perceived dysfunction and enhances self-regard. The sense of failure is restated as success and agency. Exclusion becomes inclusion when pregnancy loss is changed into a valid and growth-enhancing feminine experience.

Focus on function also implies women who have experienced pregnancy, regardless of the length, are mothers. The transform-ation to mothering and maternal-fetal attachment takes place in utero (Slade et al.; Doan and Zimerman; Mercer; Rabuzi; Rubin; Stern; Stern and Bruschweiler-Stern). Accordingly, while the women were pregnant, their bodies mothered and grew babies. The mothers' tasks changed following loss while feelings attached to mothering may have remained strong. Women can get in touch with their experience of mothering by discussing various ways they may have nurtured their unborn children. Some may have fantasized and attached to the unborn embryo or fetus. It is helpful to provide women with opportunities to discuss their sensations, possible interactions with the embryo or fetus, and their dreams. They should re-experience the good feelings they may have felt during pregnancy. This tactic is also available to women with unsuccessful attempts at pregnancy. In this case, we talk about their very real dreams about how they mothered babies in their minds. Women should see that they know what it is to feel love for an offspring, which further reduces the sense of difference from those they believe exclude them. The experience may become even more credible when women realize they may have learned lessons about nurturing they can apply in other situations. As part of the validation process, I refer to women as mothers, but only if this suits them. The designation of mother provides some women with a sense of inclusion in a desired group, and promotes healing.

Thus, the process of supporting growth is individual and includes discussing novel concepts that have relevance for the woman engaging in transformation. Empathetic and supportive listening enables women to talk, process trauma, and reframe and work out feelings impairing function. The sense of voice, inclusion and agency enhances opportunities for emotional growth. Novel cognitions may be woven in while mothers reconstruct their story. Women can focus on what they feel they did right and the lessons learned. By the same token, some may decide, because they are in control, to keep difficult moments in the narrative for now or forever. Mothers realize positive attributes, integrate strengths, acknowledge their connection to the female continuum, and realize moments of working physiology and the experience of mothering during pregnancy. They reframe how the experience of pregnancy loss makes them feel more like a woman and part of a long historical continuum of sisterhood. In my experience, women also like to speak about how they are resilient and can bounce back following loss. They may ponder how the pregnancy and/or mothering and loss affect their lives or the mothering of live children. And like me, I wonder if they may also celebrate treasured parts of the loss and recognize the special insights or skills they have gained.

Insights I have gained through genuine interactions with those who share my experience of the devastation of pregnancy loss have helped me provide a voice to silenced women. My experiences have helped me reframe exclusion into a narrative of inclusion and pride and into new way of knowing as a woman. Emotional repair is enhanced by validating the devastation associated with miscarriage and the loss of an infant while normalizing the event as an important component of a normal female physiological and emotional continuum. This model complements but does not take the place of more intensive modes of support when required. Nor will this model take away the longstanding pain. It is a mother's right to never forget, and to hold onto dreams whether or not they were ever actualized. However, focus on positive attributes concealed by culture helps women accept their pain along with the knowledge of and ability to proclaim growth, agency, and inclusion in the significant continuum of womanhood.

This chapter is dedicated to the memory of my mother Carol Joy Weinstein Epstein Z"L.

WORKS CITED

Austin-Smith, Brenda. "The Miscarriage." *Canadian Dimension*, vol. 32, no. 3, 1998, pp. 45.

Borg, Susan and Judith Lasker. *When Pregnancy Fails: Families Coping With Miscarriage, Stillbirth and Infant Death*. Beacon Press, 1982.

Brier, Norman. "Anxiety after Miscarriage: A Review of the Empirical Literature and Implications For Clinical Practice." *Birth*, vol. 31, no. 2, 2004, pp. 138-42.

Davis, Deborah, L. *Empty Cradle, Broken Heart: Surviving the Death of Your Baby*. 2nd ed. Fulcrum Publishing, 1996.

Doan, Helen, and Anona Zimerman. "Conceptualizing Prenatal Attachment: Towards a Multidimensional View." *Journal of Prenatal and Perinatal Psychology*, vol. 18, no. 2-3, 2003, pp. 109-29.

Doka, Kenneth J. "Disenfranchised Grief." *Bereavement Care*, vol. 18, no. 3, 1999, pp. 37-39.

Ellis, Albert. "The Revised ABC's of Rational-Emotive Therapy." *Journal of Rational-Emotive and Cognitive Behavior Therapy*, vol. 9, no. 3, 1991, pp. 139-72.

Epstein-Gilboa, Karen. *Systemic Interactions in Breastfeeding Families*. Doctoral Dissertation. OISE: University of Toronto, 2006.

Epstein-Gilboa, Karen. *Interaction and Relationships in Breastfeeding Families: Implications for Practice*. Hale publishing, 2009.

Epstein-Gilboa, Karen. "Breastfeeding Envy: Unresolved Patriarchal Envy and the Obstruction of Physiologically-Based Nursing Patterns." *Giving Milk*, edited by Alison Bartlett and Rhona Shaw, Demeter Press, 2010, pp. 205-21.

Epstein-Gilboa, Keren. "Maternal Ambivalence: Breastfeeding Mothers' Attempts to Resolve the Conflicting Desire to Be Close to Children and to Fulfill Western Conceptualizations of Self Worth and Equality." *Stay at Home Mothers: An International Perspective*, edited by Elizabeth Reid Boyd and Gayle Letherby, Demeter Press, 2014, pp.31-41

Geller, Pamela, et al. "Anxiety Disorders Following Miscarriage." *Journal of Clinical Psychiatry*, vol. 62, no. 6, 2001, pp. 432-38.

Hayes, Steven C., et al. "Acceptance and Commitment Therapy and Contextual Behavioral Science: Examining the Progress of a Distinctive Model of Behavioral and Cognitive Therapy." *Behavior Therapy*, vol. 44, no. 2, 2013, pp. 180-98.

Herman, Judith. *Trauma and Recovery. The Aftermath of Violence-from Domestic Abuse to Political Terror.* Basic Books, 1997.

Hsu, Min-Tao, et al. "Interpretations of Stillbirth." *Journal of Advanced Nursing*, vol. 47, no. 4, 2004, pp. 408-16.

Jordan, Judith V. *Relational-Cultural Therapy*. American Psychological Association, 2010.

Kabat-Zinn, Jon. *Coming To Our Senses: Healing Ourselves and The World through Mindfulness.* Hyperion 2004.

Karraa, Walker. *Transformed by Postpartum Depression: Women's Stories of Trauma and Growth*. Praeclarus Press, 2014.

Klein, Melanie. *Love Guilt and Reparation and Other Works: 1921-1945*. Vintage, 1998.

Klier, Claudia M., et. al. "Minor Depressive Disorder in the Context of Miscarriage." *Journal of Affective Disorders*, vol. 59, no. 1, 2000, pp. 13-21.

Lee, C., and Pamela Slade. "Miscarriage as a Traumatic Event: A Review of Literature and Implications for Intervention." *Journal of Psychosomatic Research,* vol. 40, no. 3, 1996, pp. 235-44.

Levine, Peter. *Trauma and Memory: Brain and Body in a Search for the Living Past.* North Atlantic Books, 2015.

Lok, Ingrid H., and Richard Neugebauer. "Psychological Morbidity Following Miscarriage. Best Practice and Research." *Clinical Obstetrics and Gynaecology,* vol. 21, no. 2, 1999, pp. 229-47.

Madden, Margaret, E. "The Variety of Emotional Reactions to Miscarriage." *Women and Health,* vol. 21, no. 2-3, 1994, pp. 85-104.

Malacrida, Claudia. "Complicating Mourning: The Social Economy of Perinatal Death." *Qualitative Health Research,* vol. 9, no. 4, 1999, pp. 504-19.

Martel, Sara. "Biopower and Reproductive Loss." *Cultural Studies*, vol. 28, no. 2, 2014, pp. 327-45.

Mercer, Ramona. *Becoming a Mother: Research on Maternal Identity from Rubin to the Present*. Springer, 1995.

Mor, Gil, and Ingrid Cardenas. "The Immune System in Pregnancy: A Unique Complexity." *American Journal of Reproductive Immunology*. vol. 63, no. 6, pp.425-433, 2010

Mulvihill, Aileen, and Trish Walsh. "Pregnancy Losss in Rural Ireland: An Experience of Disenfranchised Grief." *The British Journal of Social Work*, vol. 44, no. 8, 2013, pp. 2290-2306.

Northrup, Christiane. *Women's Bodies, Women's Wisdom: Creating Physical and Emotional Health and Healing*. Bantam Books, 1995.

Paloma-Castro, Olga, et al. "Nursing Diagnosis of Grieving: Content Validity in Perinatal Loss Situations." *International Journal of Nursing Knowledge*, vol. 25, no. 2, pp. 102-09, 2013.

Rabuzzi, Kathryn Allen. *Mother with Child: Transformations through Childbirth*. Indiana University Press, 1994.

Racicot, Karen, et al. "Understanding the Complexity of the Immune System during Pregnancy." *American Journal of Reproductive Immunology*, vol. 72, no. 2, 2014, pp.107-16.

Robinson, Gail Erlick. "Pregnancy Loss. Best Practice and Research." *Clinical Obstetrics and Gynaecology*, vol. 28, no. 1, 2015, pp. 169-78.

Rogers, Carl. *On Becoming a Person*. Houghton Mifflin, 1961

Rowlands, Ingrid Jean, and Christina Lee. "The Silence Was Deafening: Social and Health Support After Miscarriage." *Journal of Reproductive and Infant Psychology*, vol. 28, no. 3, 2010, pp. 274-86.

Rubin, Reva. *The Maternal Identity and the Maternal Experience*. Springer, 1984.

Shapiro, Francine. *Eye Movement Desensitization and Reprocessing: Basic Principles, Protocols and Procedures*. 2nd ed. The Guilford Press, 2001.

Slade, Arietta, et al. "The Psychology and Psychopathology of Pregnancy: Reorganization and Transformation." *Handbook of Infant Mental Health*, edited by Charles. H. Zeanah, The Guildford Press, 2009, pp. 40-58.

Solomon, Joyce. "Kaddishes Lost and Found." *Kaddish: Women's Voices*, edited by Michal Smart and Barbara Ashkenas, Urim Publications, 2013, pp. 207-08.

Stern, Daniel. *The Motherhood Constellation*. Karnac, 1998.

Stern, Daniel, and Nadia Bruschweiler-Stern. *The Birth of a Mother*. Basic Books, 1998.

Van der Kolk, Bessel. *The Body Keeps Score: Brain Mind and Body in the Healing of Trauma*. Viking, 2014.

Wojnar, Danuta, et al. "Confronting the Inevitable: A Conceptual Model of Miscarriage for Use in Clinical Practice and Research." *Death Studies*, vol. 35, no. 6, 2011, pp. 536-58.

White, Michael. *Narrative Practice: Continuing the Conversation*. Norton, 2011.

Wright, Patricia M., and Beth P. Perry. "Perinatal Loss." *International Journal of Childbirth Education*, vol. 28, no. 1, pp. 15-19.

8.
~~failing~~

j wallace skelton

As a trans person, I am used to my body failing me.

As a ~~trans~~ person, I am used to my body failing me.

As a trans person, I am used to my body ~~failing me~~.

As a trans person, I am ~~used to~~ my body ~~failing me~~.

~~As a trans person,~~ I am ~~used to~~ my body ~~failing me~~.

~~As a trans person,~~ I ~~am~~ used ~~to~~ my body ~~failing me~~.

As a trans person, I am used to ~~my body~~ failing ~~me~~.

As ~~a trans person,~~ I ~~am used to my body~~ failing ~~me~~.

~~As a trans person,~~ I am ~~used to my body failing me~~.

AS A TRANS PERSON, I AM USED TO MY BODY FAILING ME

T HIS IS THE expected narrative. This ushers in a story of puberty in the wrong direction, of breasts where the previously flat chest was preferred, of bleeding. Puberty sucked in those ways, but it also made me fuzzy, and the chest hair and facial hair was/ is delightful. My body is like me, able to excel in some areas, and shite in others.

"As a trans person, I am use to my body failing me" is a softer version of the official trans narrative: "I was trapped in the wrong body." That is not my narrative. Frankly, there are a great many people who learned to say this because it is what gender clinics and people reading trans autobiographies expect to hear. Some people feel that, but many of us do not imagine our bodies as cages. I am not trapped in my body. This is my body, and I live here, and in living here, I need to make this body a place I can thrive. I've learned to value strength, power in my limbs. I've learned to love my stamina, I've learned to come home to my imperfect flesh. In seeking to be pregnant, I felt like I needed to feel at home in my body before I could invite someone else to live in it with me. I clean the house before company comes over too, I want my home to be better for other people than it is for me alone. I wanted that in my body, too.

It's not lost on me that those uncomfortable pubertal changes, the breasts, the bleeding, are the same ones that allow me to be pregnant and grow someone new. My body's failures are productive or, at least, potentially productive. What if we can only achieve through failure? What if we need to be broken to create? In allowing myself to want, to imagine, to think about pregnancy, I also find a gentleness with my body, an acceptance of the soft parts I found hard. Failure is an ugly word for anomaly.

My mother wants to know if I miscarried because of the testosterone. It's possible other people want to ask too, but they don't. The question slams through my chest demanding to know if my body failed at pregnancy because I am trans. My mother doesn't know my medical history, doesn't know medical science, and in the absence of either, her question is built out of transphobia and fear. I hear blame. Rationally, I know pregnancies fail, not bodies, but still, self-reproach is more familiar. I don't want to blame the being that will never now be born, I don't want to blame myself, I don't want to blame at all, I just want to mourn. I don't know how to answer her question, I don't have it to lovingly strip away the assumptions and transphobia. I don't have an answer, and at that moment, I don't have a pregnancy either, and I'm angry that she has skipped on to looking for why as I am still in the throws of NO.

AS A ~~TRANS~~ PERSON, I AM USED TO MY BODY FAILING ME

After the first miscarriage, we decided we would tell people when we got pregnant. Not telling people means either you miscarry without support, or you find yourself telling people about the pregnancy and miscarriage at the same time. After the first miscarriage, we decided we would tell the people we wanted on the journey with us. If there was joy, we wanted to be able to share it, and if there was mourning, we wanted to be able to share that too, and mourn together. Not telling people I was pregnant had not protected my feelings, and it had not protected the pregnancy. It might have protected our friends from the knowledge of our miscarriage but at the cost of isolation and a denial of intimacy. The next time there were two lines, we shared our news. Miscarriage made that next pregnancy feel vulnerable. Instead of feeling pregnant, I felt "a little bit pregnant."

When this pregnancy too became one that was not going to result in a baby, we told people. I wrote about it, in part so that I did not have to talk about it all the time. In naming our miscarriage, I discovered failure is inherently part of having a body. Almost all the people I know who had tried to create babies experienced miscarriage. Some had experienced it over and over again. It was incredibly helpful to know how common this was, to mourn my loss, and their losses, to feel broken in community. It felt like there was a giant conspiracy of silence around miscarriage, and the silence had fostered shame, and blame, and guilt, and the sense that everyone else had perfect bodies that did what was wanted of them. Suddenly we were imperfect together.

AS ~~A TRANS PERSON, I AM USED TO MY BODY~~ FAILING ~~ME~~

I am not willing to allow that miscarriage is a failure of the body, but it is most certainly a failure of hope. It is, however, the very nature of hope to begin again, and to start anew.

Lest it sound like I think having a uterus is a failure, let me be clear that I think failure is part of the human condition. Our bodies do not respond to regulation as we would like. They are unruly. They break when we want them to bend, they hurt when they would rather we not. Capitalism depends on us feeling like our bodies are failures, and the weight-loss industry, the fashion industry, and the plastic surgery industry all actively work to foster that. Having a body is hard, but it is better than the alternative. I did not fail because I was trans, I failed because I had a body, and if all of us are failing, perhaps we need to let that go, and get on with being instead.

AS A TRANS PERSON, I AM USED TO MY BODY ~~FAILING ME~~

Being trans and fertility monitoring have taught me the most about my body. Both are fundamentally embodied businesses. Being trans, I studied how I move in the world and how other people move in the world. It caused me to pay attention to how other people move, and think about what behaviours I want to make muscle memories out of. Being trans makes me more aware of my breath, of my chest expanding and pushing against my binder, of the rise and fall of my lungs pushing against my ribs, and of societal expectations in a single breath. Being trans teaches me to read other's faces, to try to understand how they are reading me—is my gender intelligible to them? What does their gender literacy read on my body? I am used to my body and to its ways.

Fertility monitoring requires attention to processes I have been actively ignoring. For me, it's easier to outsource some of it. I went to the fertility clinic for monitoring because if every encounter with sperm requires travel to the United States, I needed to get the timing right. Blood work and ultrasounds seems so scientific, so more reliable that anything I can monitor at home, yet, instead of providing the answers, they teach me how to look for the signs myself. I learn to read ovulation in my body. After the second miscarriage, the fertility clinic told me after thirty days, I would bleed again, and then I should come back, and we would start the process over again. At thirty days, I read ovulation in my body, not menstruation. My body, without monitoring, without any of the talismanic behaviours, was doing the thing I had wanted every cycle. Preparing, launching, making. In my own retrospective magical thinking, I think it was because this time, there was canoeing.

AS A TRANS PERSON, I AM ~~USED TO~~ MY BODY ~~FAILING ME~~

As a feminist, my body is mine, and my fertility choices are my own damn business. Canadian fertility law, on the other hand, is not feminist, and in making choices in starting and ending pregnancy as a trans person, as a queer person, I danced on the edges of it. If you are not having sex with the person whose sperm you intend to use to create a pregnancy, Canadian law has rules about whose sperm, and how it needs to be treated. "The state has no business in the bedrooms of the nation" sounds nice, but the state remains deeply interested in what happens in your bedroom if it may involve procreation. Disallowing men who have had sex with men, even once, since 1977 to donate sperm denies reproductive choices. Does the government worry queerness is hereditary? Are they looking to prevent us passing on the gay to our theoretical children? Much of the joy in my life comes through queer and trans cultures, and I am sharing this with my children. My children, regardless of what identities they grow into, are culturally queer and culturally trans, and richer for it. Queerness is desirable.

As presented, the blood libel, this "even once since 1977," is about preventing HIV. Does the government believe what we shouted in the eighties, and nineties, the aughts, and still, that we all have AIDS? This is not what we meant. Not that all the queers have AIDS but that our society has AIDS. There is no protection in this, no "safe keeping," no option for informed consent. This is about criminalizing AIDS, criminalizing queers, and preventing possible queer children. Funny thing, now that well-medicated poz folks can have zero viral loads and now that clinics can wash sperm, there are men with HIV creating babies that are not poz. There are pregnant poz folk who are having HIV-negative babies. The law does not reflect the science or reality. It just stops queer people who make sperm from donating that sperm to make babies.

The fertility clinic said that our spuncle could undergo a full range of testing, deposit sperm, have it frozen, and six months later, if a second round of testing said he did not present me with any health risks, I could try to get knocked-up using his spermsicles. We would have to pay for the testing, sperm washing, storage, testing, and then probably insemination because thawed sperm is just not as mobile as fresh. The government wants queers to pay the queer tax, and I was not fucking having it. Still, at forty, with two miscarriages behind me, I wanted to increase our chances of success. So, like queer culture, I gave the middle finger to the law. Telling you more would have legal risks for me, the person who helped me, and my family, so I'm going to leave it there. I will say that it felt profoundly feminist. I thought about groups in the seventies who engaged in home menstrual extraction, and the promise of "Our Bodies, Ourselves." I would offer the same assistance to other people if it would not mean risking being charged with "practicing medicine without a license."

~~AS A TRANS PERSON,~~ I AM ~~USED TO~~ MY BODY ~~FAILING ME~~

I am my body. We are inseparable. But I am also a hybrid, a chimera. Increasingly, science recognizes fetal cells cross into the gestational parent, living in us, becoming part of us. This is true for the two children that I birthed and for the two pregnancies that did not result in babies. My body is mine, and my pregnancies are written into it. I love the idea that this makes pregnancy into a trans-ing of the body. I was just me, and now, now I always have company in my body, cells that I made and are not me. As the two I birthed grow, and I know more and more about them, I imagine their personalities in their cells I still carry. I don't get to know anymore about the two that never came into being, but I imagine their cells still within me. We are all intimate. The body does not discriminate between the ones who arrived and the ones who did not, and I have a tiny chorus of others inside me. Sometimes I imagine this a genetic photo album inside me, in my blood. I love knowing the traces of even the ones that never arrived get to come home in my body. Neither miscarriage was a total loss, my body continues to sustain tiny parts. I love that my body remembers.

~~AS A TRANS PERSON,~~ I ~~AM~~ USED ~~TO~~ MY BODY ~~FAILING ME~~

We all use our bodies. I used mine for pregnancy and for nursing, and now I am reshaping my body for other uses. Being trans encourages me to think about how I want to use my body and what changes I might make. I am in constant renovation. I use surgery, hormones, food and exercise, love and touch to remake this body. How do you use your body? What tools are you using to change it? Permanently? For today? For Halloween? I move between being my body and using my body, and try to foster the possibilities in both.

AS A TRANS PERSON, I AM USED TO ~~MY BODY~~ FAILING ~~ME~~

And as such, it was almost a surprise when the next pregnancy continued. Continued, and lasted, and shaped both me and a new person. Everyone is different. It's true for pregnancy, and birth, and children. I had imagined the first pregnancy ending with a birth in a pool in our living room. If that was the goal, I failed, so I shifted the goal. That baby arrived in hospital, through surgery, and none of that was a failure. The notion of failure is what failed. The second and third pregnancies were not my failures, even as they were failures of pregnancy. Failures-not-failures at the same time. In this last pregnancy, I expected more failure, I'm fat, I was over forty, and I was told to expect failure. I expected miscarriage, and that failure, ultimately failed. I expected surgery and failed to need it. Expecting failure allowed me to feel ready for more possibilities. Which perhaps is the best possible preparation for parenthood, as long as it is also coupled with the expectation of success. Expect failure. Expect success. Prepare for both.

~~AS A TRANS PERSON, I AM USED TO MY BODY FAILING ME~~

I am.
I am.
I am.
You are too.
And you contain your own poetry.

9.
Fatphobia, Pregnancy Loss, and My Hegemonic Imagination

A Story of Two Abortions

EMILY R. M. LIND

Throughout human history, most women have not chosen their pregnancies.—Caroline Lundquist (136)

When pregnancy is not chosen, not achieved, fails or ends unhappily, the life course appears disrupted and the social illusion of reproductive control—where one exists—is shattered.—Sarah Earle et al. (3)

WHAT DOES IT MEAN to choose a pregnancy, and who is the subject who chooses? If we take seriously the postmodern premise that subjectivity is unfixed, fluid, or otherwise multiply positioned, then can the same be said for the reproductive choices made and remade over the course of a lifetime? This personal essay considers abortion as a social experience, and highlights the implications that making the choice to terminate pregnancies had on my shifting sense of self. I consider the epistemological implications of pregnancy loss and what I learned about my social location from my experience of abortion.

As a feminist educator, my course syllabi often read like top ten lists of social justice issues: "abortion rights" one week, "compulsory heterosexuality" the next, "understanding rape culture," and so on. In my experience, the dynamics of the classroom during any given week mirror the dynamics of public discourse about the issue we are studying. Lived experience can be used in the classroom to empower students to mine their stories to contribute to theoretical discussions. I have witnessed queer students leaning confidently on their experience of heterosexism when elaborating on the myriad ways compulsory heterosexuality affects our social world. Similarly, I have watched as white students struggle to articulate their experience of whiteness or colonialism in a white supremacist, settler colonial society. My experience of teaching students to recognize the relationships between power and identity is that some identities are more easily articulated than others. Silence, I often remind my students, is a central axis through which power expresses itself.

Recently, in anticipation of a class that was scheduled to discuss abortion rights, I received several tentative emails from students: "Dear Professor, I'm nervous about attending the upcoming class"; or "Dear Professor, please don't call on me. I'm going through issues related to the class topic this week." My students emailed to contextualize their upcoming silence. Through their nervous warnings, they applied the lessons I had taught them in class. They were identifying their silence as related to their lived experience, and they were calling my attention to it. Most importantly, they reminded me that the study of abortion cannot be limited to a series of facts and significant historical events. Abortion is of course a social issue, and as I prepared my lecture, I realized that my students' honesty was more than just feedback. Their disclosures extended an invitation to me to address my own relationship to abortion in the context of studying abortion access.

This personal essay is an attempt to consider abortion as a social experience—to expand the conceptual frame of reference used in academic and social understandings of the circumstances surrounding abortion, in particular as it relates to parental subjectivity. My essay is a contribution to the literature on abortion as a social experience as opposed to a moral dilemma (Purcell 593). By supporting an expanded conceptual framework for understanding abortion experiences, I hope that abortion will cease to be disavowed as an essential part of the maternal experience (Hudson 50).

MY STORY

In my mid-twenties, I had two abortions, twenty-two months apart. The first time I became pregnant, I was twenty-five years old, and three weeks into my first professional job. My partner and I were fighting one morning. In an effort to quickly deescalate and leave for work, I dismissed my stake in the argument, and said, "don't even listen to me. I feel really premenstrual and I must be sensitive." He eyed me with nervous suspicion and looked in his calendar. "You sure you're only premenstrual?" We looked at each other for a long, stunned, ten seconds. "Let's hope," I said. "I'll talk to you after work." By 10:00 a.m., I had taken a pregnancy test: the "positive" line marched defiantly across the result screen as I sat stunned in the staff bathroom.

I instantly went numb. My body felt empty and flushed with panic. In that moment, I felt time accelerate at an uncomfortable pace. For years, I had been anticipating my entry into parenthood. It was one of the few things I felt no ambivalence about. I yearned to parent, looked forward to pregnancy, and did not want to delay family planning much longer. Yet *this* version of pregnancy, *this* catapult into maternity felt wholly, painfully, and urgently *wrong*. It would take me years before I could articulate why, years I would spend confused and muddled in a mix of relief and regret at how the story played out. Staring at the positive pregnancy test in a bathroom stall that summer morning, an inarguable feeling persisted: this was not a trajectory I could allow to continue uninterrupted.

I held onto the information that I was pregnant for a week, hardly telling anyone. My partner sat passively by, telling me it was my choice to make. Maybe he suggested he'd support me either way, but that support didn't come with any significant strategizing or consideration for arguments in either direction. I hated that it was my choice to make. I resented him for being able to look noble by doing nothing. What stunned me was the raging bitterness that it *was* my choice to make, in many ways a dilemma brought to me, through my body, through our collective actions, which *I* now needed to shoulder alone. The notion that the decision was my choice (and mine alone) echoed in both my and my partner's consciousness, as a rebuttal to generations of paternalistic logic and legislation. For as long as I could remember, I had been told reproductive choice was mine to claim. For as long as I could remember, I was taught that women's liberation was bound to the right to choose. No amount of fluency in second-wave political slogans prepared me for the intricacies of my decision to terminate my first pregnancy. Nothing felt less liberating than feeling trapped in my own body and confronting a contradiction for which I had no preparation: my decision to abort would have little to do with my desire to parent.

I was certain I wanted to parent. I was certain I was old enough to parent. But carrying that particular pregnancy to term would lock me in a set of relationships I worried would kill me: a job I hated, a deteriorating relationship, and a spontaneous rewriting of my assumed life narrative. In this way, the first lesson I learned from abortion was that the decision to carry a pregnancy to term intersects with all facets of a person's social location.

Although I was surprised to find myself trapped in my own body upon discovering I was pregnant, I was more surprised to realize how familiar this feeling felt. As a fat woman, my social experience of the world is mitigated by the persistent micro and macro aggressions of fatphobia. My body's social legitimacy is undermined on a daily basis by the sociomedical assumptions projected onto it. The stories I tell are painful but common: I have been accused of poor eating habits because of my size; looked upon with suspicion in gyms and fitness facilities as though my body must necessarily be inactive; and, of course, excluded from purchasing clothing in conventional stores. Fatphobia characterizes fat bodies as unhealthy, unattractive, inactive, and unnatural. Significantly, these characterizations are inherently temporal ideas: the fat body is imagined to be the *consequence* of poor choices, rather than simply a natural size variant of the human condition. Fatphobia imagines fat bodies as future-thin bodies and awaits corrective measures—such as food restriction, strategic exercise, or medical intervention—to redeem the offending adipose. Fat, in this sense, is never validated as an unproblematic present in the cultural imagination, only a current crisis to be redeemed in the future, to correct an aberrant past (Lind et al.). Fatphobic discourse relies on an anticipatory logic—waiting for life to get better. In this way, fatphobia and pronatalism share an investment in an imagined future self. When I found out I was both fat and pregnant, I found myself overwhelmed with trying to make sense of my body and its reproductive capacity. Could I accept that my body was capable of carrying a pregnancy? Was

I allowed to willingly pursue a reproductive future in the body I inhabited? Wasn't this body of mine a symbol of failure? How could I move forward in my life with a fat body?

Until the day I first found out I was pregnant, I spent my life anticipating finding out I was pregnant in a joyful context. I expected it to be uncomplicated. I never really considered feeling half-ready. I expected to plan a pregnancy at the appropriate time, and that somehow I'd just *know* I was ready. The "just knowing," I assumed, would follow after earning a decent and regular income, after formalizing a romantic relationship, perhaps even after buying a house. While considering whether or not to carry my first pregnancy to term, I was consumed with confusion: yes, I was in a relationship, one I once thought was a relationship I would work to keep permanently in my life, but now I wasn't so sure. And yes, I had a good job, with a strong possibility of economic advancement. But I hated going to work every day. Beyond these conventional markers of middle-class readiness, however, was a seething, persistent worry I was too shy to name out loud: I was fat. I was fat, and had always been fat, and because of that, I always assumed that I had to lose weight before beginning my adult life in earnest. I had also assumed my fat body was broken, incapable or somehow not allowed to be pregnant until it appeared socially valid. To find out I was pregnant in these circumstances was never how I expected it to look. I expected to need to earn more money prior to parenting. I expected to have a different kind of relationship. And I expected living the life I had always hoped for would require that I starve myself thin before it could possibly happen.

That imagined future was marked by an expectation of a normative life course, one where parenthood would follow the establishment of a professional career in the context of a formalized, monogamous relationship. By confronting the realities of an unplanned pregnancy, I confronted the incoherence of my own story. By incoherent, I mean the conflicts and ruptures my story presented to the conventional narrative model of how life should unfold. My unplanned pregnancy called into question the assumed inevitability of bourgeois time. By not adhering to the bourgeois order of things, my life was becoming something unrecognizable to my young mind. In this way, my experience of pregnancy was what Iris Marion Young has characterized as a decentred subjectivity, a sense of "myself in the mode of not being myself" (qtd. in Lundquist 138). I ached to experience the kind of pregnancy I had grown up believing I would have—one benefiting from the social legitimacy promised by wealth and relationship status.

I was so young. I hoped I still had time to get my life back on track. I needed to get rid of the pregnancy because it threatened my sense of self and my sense of my own future. In that way, my pregnancy became like Kristeva's concept of the abject—physical "secretions ... that threatened the subject's 'own' proper body and therefore had to be expelled ... in more abstract terms, [the abject] is everything that threatens a stable subject position, disturbs social reason or messes with the communal consensus that underpins social order" (qtd. in Hudson 42). My body was no longer intelligible to me as a stable site; my sense of my own future was threatened by my pregnant state.

In order to rescue my sense of self, I decided to terminate my first pregnancy.

I remembered the name of a feminist reproductive health clinic from one of my undergraduate women's studies classes, and made the call. A small army of feminist nurses guided me through the process, and patiently outlined the choices available to me. At only seven-weeks pregnant, I was eligible for a medical abortion. I took a few days off of work, passed the tissue at home, recovered easily, and later felt proud of my decision and the services I was able to access without significant barriers. Later, I would tell friends I felt no regret about the procedure. I felt empowered; I had claimed my own life through that choice. I was lucky to have a prochoice family and social circle. My choice was never stigmatized, and many in my network agreed with me when I said I didn't feel economically ready to become a parent. By terminating my pregnancy, I was able to return to a mythical life trajectory still on track.

Twenty-one months later, my relationship remained unhappy, and I had decided to leave. The stress of finishing my master's degree, my grandmother's death, and my ailing relationship contributed to my lack of alarm when my period stopped coming regularly each month. During my annual physical, my doctor asked when my last period had been. I told her six weeks previous, but I had been bleeding every eight. She told me she'd throw in a pregnancy test for good measure. I shrugged and reminded her that I was certain I wasn't pregnant. She told me to come back in three weeks for test results.

Three weeks later, my doctor read my test results: negative for many things, including pregnancy and diabetes. "How's your period?" she asked. "I haven't gotten it yet." I explained, matter-of-factly. I watched her push the file to the back of her desk. "Alright," she said. "It's time we had a talk. Your body is likely in a diabetic state, and it's possible you have polycystic ovarian syndrome. Conceiving children is going to be very difficult, if it happens at all. You need to stop eating carb-rich foods: fettuccine alfredo, burgers and fries ... have you seen the carbohydrate content of a hamburger and fries lately? It's insane!"

"But I don't eat that stuff," I mumbled meekly, "at least not regularly. I can't even tell you when I last had fettuccine alfredo. And I might have one burger a month."

"You must be eating it" she said, "Look at you. Something's going on."

Indeed, something was.

I spent the next month wandering around in a fog of depression and anxiety. Her off-the-cuff diagnosis confirmed my worse fears: my body *was* broken. I *was* too fat to conceive. My size was only intelligible as a consequence of pathologized food choices, as opposed to the beauty of my genetic makeup. I found myself terrified to eat each day, convinced I had an eating disorder I couldn't recognize. I became convinced that I couldn't trust my hunger cues or metabolism.

Two weeks later, I curiously bought myself a pregnancy test. I again saw the "positive" line appear rapidly in the results window. I had been accepted into my doctoral program two days earlier. Once again, I confronted two competing futures: an unplanned pregnancy with a partner I had doubts about, or the promise of upper-middle-class mobility if I delayed family planning further.

I called the abortion clinic. My lack of trauma from my first abortion informed my confidence about booking a second abortion. At the clinic, I would discover I was eleven-weeks pregnant.

I had been pregnant when I was told I would have a hard time conceiving children. I was pregnant when I was told I was likely diabetic. I was pregnant when I was accused of being fat because of a fetish for burgers and fettuccine alfredo. I was pregnant while too nervous to eat. Pregnant while worrying I would never become a parent because my body was too broken, too fat, too gross.

I walked around numb for months.

I now understand that I was mourning my decision to terminate my second pregnancy, not because I regretted it but because I regretted the fact that abortion presented itself once again as the best option. I was mourning the extent to which fatphobia had divorced me from my physical self—both in my incapacity to recognize the symptoms of early pregnancy and in my misguided belief I was incapable of being pregnant at all. I mourned the fact that had I been in a different relationship, I may well have carried the pregnancy to term. I had once again confronted a "split subjectivity" in my experience of pregnancy, one that positioned me in relation to my pregnancy as a "subject and some unwanted or menacing object, some less than human, perhaps monstrous creature" (Lundquist 141). To rescue my sense of self, I needed to once again terminate my pregnancy. The self I rescued, however, was not a unified sense of self, but rather the promise of a unified sense of self. I terminated my pregnancy with the hope that in the future, I would be able to plan and choose a pregnancy I wanted to carry to term.

IMPLICATIONS OF MY STORY

Understanding myself and making sense of my story from these losses has compelled me to understand more clearly the extent to which my body and my sexuality are embedded in my class status. That my choice was largely informed by a desire to later follow a less scrutinized, more socially acceptable path to parenthood demonstrates how intimately connected my experiences of pregnancy were to a desire to assimilate into upper-middle-class conventions. My choice to terminate did not reflect an unwillingness to parent but an unwillingness to spontaneously reject a trajectory I had never before questioned. By carrying my pregnancies to term, I felt as though I would be preventing myself from creating a normative family model, and at the time, that felt too threatening. Tragically, I also believed my body was broken, a narrative reinforced by my doctor's fatphobic assumptions. Discovering I had been pregnant the whole time I fretted about whether I was unconsciously bingeing on fettuccine alfredo forced me to confront the validity of my own existence. I was not fat because of disordered eating or a pathological diagnosis; I was fat because my body is fat. Not because it is yearning to be thin or awaiting a transformative diet regimen, but because this is who I am.

These revelations conspire to reveal some of the hidden operations of whiteness. I understand whiteness to be a social construct that relies on invisibility by masquerading as social conformity.[1] So-called white people are encouraged by white supremacy to think of themselves as race neutral, unmarked, or invisible. The boundaries of whiteness are policed by categories of respectability. Markedness threatens one's belonging in white sensibilities, and can take the shape of working-class affectations, fatness, so-called ethnic food, behaviour, dress, or smell—all aspects of identity quietly subdued in order to pass as white. My decision to terminate to remain invisible as well as the subsequent grappling and grieving of these particular experiences of pregnancy loss constitute the labour of whiteness. I have worked at remaining invisible and have hidden this narrative from my life, my teaching, and my activism in order to keep it invisible. The invisibility rewards me with a coherent life narrative, one where I was able to complete a PhD prior to becoming a parent. Terminating my first two pregnancies helped me to avoid the lamentation that I was trapped in a dysfunctional relationship for the sake of the kids. These possibilities allow social categories to remain flexible, a constitutive staple of white privilege.

MUSINGS ABOUT A FEMINIST EPISTEMOLOGY OF LOSS

What I know from what I have lost is that the potential for a coherent self is part of the hegemonic imagination. The myth of the coherent self was never going to be a source of empowerment for me, as much as it promised to be the source of social legitimacy. In order to choose my future, I would need to heal my relationship to my body, recognize it not as a broken mass of failed food choices but as a gorgeous reflection of who I am.

My experience of pregnancy loss is characterized by the willful act to lose. I willed myself to lose the chance to continue carrying my first two pregnancies. There are moments where I regret my abortions. In those moments of regret, I am forced to confront the fact that such regret assumes that I would have had a normative pregnancy and a normative child. My regret is a form of disavowal, as it denies the possibilities my pregnancies could have ended in miscarriage or stillbirth. In other words: my regret assumes my abortion caused a pregnancy loss I would have otherwise been spared, and that is simply unknowable. In this way, a feminist epistemology of loss must acknowledge the epistemic limits left in the wake of loss. Rather than characterizing pregnancy loss as the loss of an otherwise perfect pregnancy, I find greater possibilities in a framework acknowledging loss as constitutive of "a more fluid self capable of bearing a much more porous relationship to another" (Bracken 80).

ENDNOTE

[1]This premise for the study of whiteness is informed in particular by chapter four, "Our Bodies Are Not Ourselves: Tranny Guys and the Racialized Politics of Incoherence" of Jean Bobby Noble's *Sons of the Movement* (2006).

WORKS CITED

Bracken, Claire. "Grounded Futurity: Time and Subjectivity in Lisa Baraister's *Maternal Encounters.*" *Studies in Gender and Sexuality*, vol. 13, no. 2, 2012, pp. 80-84.

Earle, Sarah, et al. "The Social Dimensions of Reproductive Loss." *Practising Midwife*, vol. 10, no. 6, 2007, pp. 28-34.

Hudson, Kirsten. "Taste My Sorrow: Caught Horribly, Somewhere, Between the Pregnant and the Maternal." *Performance Research*, vol. 19, no. 1, 2014, pp. 41-51.

Lind, Emily R.M., et al. "Re-conceptualizing Temporality in and through Multi-Media Storytelling: Making Time with *Through*

Thick and Thin." *Fat Studies: An Interdisciplinary Journal of Body Weight and Society*, vol. 7, no. 2 (Forthcoming Spring 2018).

Lundquist, Caroline. "Being Torn: Towards a Phenomenology of Unwanted Pregnancy." *Hypatia*, vol. 23, no. 3, 2008, pp. 136-55.

Noble, Jean Bobby. *Sons of the Movement: FtMs Risking Incoherence on a Post-Queer Cultural Landscape*. Women's Press, 2006.

Purcell, Carrie. "The Sociology of Women's Abortion Experiences: Recent Research and Future Directions." *Sociology Compass*, vol. 9, no. 7, 2015, pp. 585-96.

10.
Missed Miscarriage

ROBIN SILBERGLEID

—for A

1.

I LOST MY first child three times.

First: in the sonogram room, with that awful Anne Geddes calendar on the wall, babies sprouting from vegetables and fruits. For months, its hyper-fecundity mocked me, the fertility patient, waiting cross-legged under a paper sheet. Then, the one I came to think of as Dr. Pretty waved his magic wand between my legs and poof, no baby, just a fluid-filled sac. My own doctor said, in her kind way, "it's not over until it's over, it might be hiding up against the sac wall, we'll look again in a few days." She eased me into loss the way I imagined she might deliver a child into the world, hands ready, open and gloved. She knew my body's work would be hard; she was prepared. I stopped taking the supplementary progesterone intended to support early pregnancy and waited for the blood that never came. That would be easier and less risky, the doctor explained, than undergoing surgery. So after a month, in a desperate attempt to allow my body to expel the tissue on its own, she ordered a shot of chemo—I had to sign a waiver saying I understood the drug could cause birth defects—and sent me home with a box of Kleenex and a list of warning signs of liver failure. After two more weeks, she donned blue scrubs and dilated my cervix, then suctioned and scraped my uterus until nothing was left of the pregnancy I so much wanted. I spent the next two nights curled on the bathroom floor in what I came to understand was labour, giving birth to berries of blood instead of the boy I named Benjamin Matthew in the long weeks before dilation and curettage (D&C).

I lost my first child three times. That is, I experienced loss over and over again. For me, miscarriage was not the single definitive moment both conventional wisdom and biomedical narratives would have us believe. It was a long process, emotionally and physically. I wanted to be pregnant; my uterus fought hard.

The medical diagnosis for this condition is "missed miscarriage," or, really, "missed abortion,"—a term horrifying in its connotation, like a woman who skipped a prearranged appointment to terminate a pregnancy. It's an inevitable miscarriage, a pregnancy that's clearly not viable, although the body doesn't recognize and expel it. A doctor performs a D&C or similar procedure to end the pregnancy that really ended earlier. In my case, after the operation, the doctor asked if I was stubborn, as my body still clung to this child that would never come to be. Even after all those long weeks, my cervix showed no evidence it wanted to let this baby go. I'd like to think I wanted him so much that my hormones were overcome with desire.

There was no word to express my love for him, just as there was no word to convey his loss. I read everything I could find—articles in medical journals, posts in online forums, the self-help guides at Barnes and Noble. Once, I had written a dissertation on the unrepresentability of loss in contemporary literature—the lack of adequate language for communicating trauma, both personal and cultural, and the failure of traditional narrative forms. Now, in the thick of miscarriage, I experienced it. The process was not linear but circular; my experience existed separate from and tethered to the diagnostic codes used to label it.

In some sense, all miscarriages are missed miscarriages, in that there's a delay between the death of the embryo or fetus and its expulsion from the body. It's the latter that the woman experiences as miscarriage, the termination of pregnancy, either through natural means or medical intervention. Yet it is also a phenomenon that once appeared to be much less frequent than it is now. That we know about missed miscarriage, that so many women I know have experienced one, has to do with the increase of sonographic monitoring in early pregnancy, as Linda Layne discusses in *Motherhood Lost*. I learned my miscarriage was inevitable at a mere seven weeks, when the heartbeat should be detected, and my D&C wasn't scheduled until almost twelve weeks, the end of the first trimester. If I hadn't undergone fertility treatment and had serial sonograms from beginning at five weeks, I would have assumed that everything was fine. I had six positive home pregnancy tests. I was nauseated. I was dizzy. And I was gaining weight like crazy.

When did the pregnancy end? Was it moments after conception? Was it when my doctor couldn't find a heartbeat? Was it after the shot of methotrexate when my hormone level finally stopped rising? Or at eleven weeks and four days when the doctor opened me on the table? For more than a month, I was pregnant but not carrying a child. It was a horrifying liminal space, my abdomen swollen with fluid and placental tissue. I felt pregnant. I craved turkey sandwiches and chocolate cake. I went to bed early and slept hard. Even the nurse at the doctor's office said "you are very pregnant," knowing full well my gestation wouldn't have a happy ending.

2.

My diagnosis was missed miscarriage, but that wasn't the miscarriage I missed. I experienced every minute of it, from the absence of the embryo on the sonogram to the blood on the bathroom floor. For weeks, a dark-haired boy followed me wherever I went, begging for French toast; like Toni Morrison's character Beloved, he was to me the incarnation of desire, the melancholic object I had once written about in my dissertation. I opted to have spinal rather than general anesthesia, in a cruel parody of childbirth, because I wanted to know the moment of loss. If my experience had been ongoing, it was not until the moment she removed the tissue that my body would finally recognize it was no longer pregnant. My poor doctor opened her mouth aghast—I don't think she has ever or since performed a D&C on a woman who was completely cognizant—and even though I dreamed about it for months (the sound of suction, the procession of the gurney, the dead weight of my toes) if I had to do it again, I'd make the same choice. I kept the bracelet from the hospital alongside my home pregnancy test. I needed proof.

No, the miscarriage I missed was the one I'll never know I experienced because I'll never know if I was really pregnant.

A chemical pregnancy refers to a pregnancy detected through hormone testing. It is a pregnancy that ends before sonographic detection of a gestational sac, a procedure that can be done as early as three weeks after conception. Without early pregnancy testing, either at the doctor's office or in the home (thanks to First Response), many women in this situation wouldn't even know they were pregnant. But to those who experience chemical pregnancies, "miscarriage" becomes a word to pin to loss, a word the clinical terminology evades. *The Oxford English Dictionary* describes miscarriage as "a failure," "a mishap or disaster," and "the spontaneous expulsion of a fetus from the womb before it is viable." Such language marks the experience as visceral, tangible, tragic. And, in terms of pregnancy, it seems, rarely used before the twentieth century to mark the loss of a baby.

What is the word for a pregnancy that is lost before it is even found? I have heard women talk about believing they were pregnant and insisting, based on symptoms, that they must have had a very early miscarriage when the test results come back negative. For a woman who wants a child, there's something easier to acknowledge about the loss of a pregnancy than the lack of pregnancy altogether. It's a miscarriage that is longed for, that is missed.

Sometimes I think that's what happened to me almost two years before the tests said I was pregnant. Even now, after a miscarriage and a successful pregnancy, I don't have the language to explain what happened, and I never told this theory to my doctor, even though our relationship was one of mutual respect. I just explained my symptoms—vaginal hemorrhaging and expelling blood clots the size of my future daughter's hands—said I was worried about hormone levels and let her check me out. I've never experienced anything like it before or since, but the closest I came was those two unfathomable nights after my D&C. It's the worst pain I've ever felt, other than nineteen hours into Pitocin-induced labour.

And the only other times I've been that nauseated and starving all at once I have indeed been pregnant. It would be easier, I think, if I could say I've had two miscarriages. Instead I have an experience that makes no biological sense to me and that I can't really explain to anyone else, even a well-meaning reproductive endocrinologist. I know it would make me sound crazy. I never had a missed period. I never had a positive pregnancy test. But something happened to me that I cannot deny. Who and what do I trust to explain this experience? My desire and intuition? My body? The doctor with her diagnostic codes, putting a number to an experience I had fundamentally alone? The truth is multiple and between.

When this—whatever it was—happened, I was desperate for a child. I'd gone off the pill, stopped taking prophylactic migraine medication and started taking prenatal vitamins, and hoped a few well-timed rounds with my on-again, off-again lover would do the trick. About a month after our last on-again encounter, I felt nauseated. The smell of garlic made me wretch. I craved greasy eggs and bacon. My period was late but not late enough, and two home tests said it was nothing doing. That was January. In April, my best friend gave birth to a son, and I spent several days expelling blood clots in my bathtub.

These are the experiences that no one ever tells you about when you get the "you're a woman now" talk with your mother and the rest of your fifth-grade class. The true stories of women's bodies, decades after Virginia Woolf, remain largely untold. And I'm so tired of silent sorrow.

I want to tell someone about the night I smashed mug after mug on the concrete floor of my patio. I want to tell someone about the day the nurse at the clinic put her hand on my belly and asked if I'd gained weight. I want to tell someone about watching Salma Hayek's *Frida* miscarry on screen and wondering if that's how it would happen to me. But, really, who wants to listen? The stories of women's bodies are not supposed to be told. We cramp. We bleed. We cry. And we do it, largely, alone.

Did I lose a child that night in the bathtub? Or did I bleed a metaphor?

You can't talk to people about a miscarriage unless you've told them you're pregnant. And even then, most women of childbearing age don't want to hear just how frequently pregnancy loss happens. And other women who've been through miscarriage, well, many of them don't want to hear about it either. A woman I know—I don't think I can consider her any longer a friend—who had suffered from a miscarriage more than a decade before became enraged with me when I attempted to confide in her about mine. She wrote about it constantly in stories and poems. It was an experience that haunted her. And once I thought the fact that we were both childless was the basis of our friendship, at least in part. What I didn't know—and I am truly sorry—is that she didn't want to talk about it. She didn't want to hear about it. She didn't want to be faced with someone who mirrored back some of the most painful moments of her life. She accused me of being insensitive, of saying that my own grief mattered more than hers. It certainly didn't matter more—I cannot imagine what she went through, losing a child she never expected to have in the first place—but it hadn't occurred to me that old festering grief might be just as raw as new grief. But if you can't tell one of your best friends about miscarriage, to whom can you speak? When I lost my first child, I lost one of my dearest friends. What I have come to understand is that she lost a dream, as well as some tissue, and I'm not sure we ever get over lost dreams.

3.

Now, almost three years, a pregnancy, and a nineteen-month-old later, I find myself astonished to admit I miss those miscarriage days. I have never been more myself, raw smashed-glass emotion, and I have never been so complete with emptiness and desire. Now, with a toddler running up and down the hall in thick-soled shoes, there is little time to think, let alone take to bed with sorrow, Vicodin, and a four-hundred-page novel. And after the blood and the cramping and the self-pity, I put on an old mix tape ("Manic Depression, 1995," an ode to my first year of grad school) and danced. I walked miles on the treadmill. I wrote poem after poem and even now I think it's some of my best work. I was self-indulgent, in the sense that I focused on me. Grieving. Getting my life together. And trying again.

These days I am more at peace than I have ever been. Thankfully, I'm done with the pills and injections and sonograms, what a friend called "the fertility nonsense." But I don't know if I would cherish my daughter this way if I hadn't lost my son. I don't think about him as much these days, but with the nights getting longer and the days getting cooler, I feel him with me again, growing, this little preschooler with a red shirt and a satchel. He comes to me in those quiet moments when the baby is asleep, the dishes are done, and the student papers are tucked away. He is as real to me as the nights I laboured to lose him. Over and over again.

WORKS CITED

Layne, Linda. *Motherhood Lost: A Feminist Account of Pregnancy Loss in America*. Routledge, 2002.

"Miscarriage." *Oxford English Dictionary*, 2017, en.oxforddictionaries.com/definition/miscarriage. Accessed 14 Sept. 2017.

11.
Full-Term Baby Loss

A How-To Guide for Mothers

RACHEL O'DONNELL

BEGINNINGS

WHEN YOU FIND OUT you are pregnant, call your best friend. Say: "I thought I was, but the first blood test came back negative!" Think: they really spring it on you, this whole pregnancy thing. Say to her, with a mild groan: "I am already eight weeks along." She laughs because she has had her baby for two years now.

"Don't worry," she says. "This is why babies take nine months to cook. You have plenty of time to get used to the idea."

So you try. Walk up and down the street, a belly proudly displayed in front of you, a womanly being with thick hair and clear skin who responds to questions with motherly charm. The questions are easy: "When are you due?" and "Is this your first?" and "Do you know if it's a boy or a girl?" Answer each with a toothy smile. Become a lover of small clothing, doula cooperatives, and wooden baby toys. Walk confidently like a grown-up and a mother, someone who is responsible for someone else.

Order decaffeinated coffee, swear off soft cheese, and heat all your food until the boiling point. Throw up in the mornings and sometimes in the afternoons. Make kale salads and take your daily tablets of DHA with acceptable herbal teas. Refuse to use the microwave. Pick out a house with multiple bedrooms, and on moving day, do not lift any heavy boxes. Research front baby carriers, back baby carriers, jogging strollers, and nursing bras. Interview pediatricians. Go to the baby store and register for important things: a set of cloth diapers and wipes, an organic changing pad cover.

Ask questions and take notes: what is that thing that fits snuggly over the car seat and why do you need it? Do you go to La Leche meetings before or after the baby comes? You are given a car seat and a bassinet. These are the things you will need.

When a classmate pours you a beer to celebrate your successful qualifying exams, turn it down. Order sparkling water instead. Think: everyone noticed you did not drink it, and with your obvious weight gain and disappearing waist, everyone knows. Later, on the subway, say to them all: "I am pregnant."

They turn to you and smile. "Good for you!" they say, but what they really mean is how in the world will you have a baby and finish your dissertation? Start sweating. You yourself do not know the answer.

On Saturdays, go to yard sales and pick out gender-neutral clothes: a yellow footie pajama set printed with ducks, a white fuzzy zipper suit for the cold.

At the midwife's office, drink a surgery substance and flip through parenting magazines as you wait for two hours to pass. Lie down and listen to the heartbeat through the fetoscope. Watch the spinning centrifuge determine your iron levels.

Take afternoon naps and learn to sleep on your side. Buy more pillows. Go to prenatal yoga classes and lean back gently on the bolster, interlacing your fingers and placing them on your belly with your eyes closed and the lights dimmed. When the instructor tells you to imagine the life growing inside of you, feel the life hiccup and kick your hand.

ENDINGS

Your first maternity clothes are a borrowed pair of jeans with an elastic band, and you are wearing them again, at the end, when your water breaks in the mall and soaks you to your feet. That day, the midwife comes and listens again to the heartbeat. You rest again on your side, wait for contractions to get stronger, and wash the soaked jeans.

Soon, the midwife returns and cannot find the heartbeat. Where did it go? It was just there. Watch her listen again. And again. She takes the fetoscope out of her ears one side at a time. Watch her mouth moving. Something about going to the hospital, should be able to find it, going to double check. Say: "I want the baby." The midwife looks at you with a sad face. "I know," she says.

Get in the car and fasten your seatbelt. Look over at your husband and say: "There is a dead baby inside me." You don't know how you manage to say this to your husband so matter-of-factly, and later, you will remember this as a moment in which you did not yet understand. You somehow thought the baby would still appear.

You are cold in the car in your pajamas. Park on the roof of the hospital and walk from the snowy parking lot through a heavy door. This is all you will remember later. How long was the trip to the hospital? Did you talk to your husband and the midwife on the way? What would you have said?

Walk down some stairs and into a brightly lit corridor and through some special door with a buzzer. Everyone in blue oversized jackets stares as you as you lie down on the table. Watch as they put gel on your giant belly and start the ultrasound, the wand moving over and over and over.

Stare up at the lights and then turn your head to the left, where there is a large window. It is still snowing. A new doctor comes in and presses harder with the probe. You stare to the left without blinking until he says your name. He asked the midwife what it is and that is how he knows. Again he says your name. Again he says it. You cannot look at him because you know what he will say and then finally you turn your head and see his head covered in a paper cap and his blue scrubs and his kind face says it: I cannot find a heartbeat. He says your name again because you have looked away from his face and back up to the lights.

Say quietly and disgraced: "Why did the baby die?"

Hear the pity in his voice before he speaks. "I don't know."

After that, after the news has been revealed and you are assumed to understand it, there is a lot of quick movement and noise. Hear words like IVs and morphine drips. People move in and out of the room, and there is discussion of the changing of shifts.

You wait and wait and wait for it to end. There is only that one kind doctor, and every time someone appears you have not seen before, ask what time the nice one will be back. Think: why did he leave without letting you know?

At night, you sleep on your side and your husband sleeps in the folding chair next to you and holds your hand. When you get up to use the bathroom, do not look in the mirror.

When the midwife comes back into the room and reports that she has called your parents like you asked her to, realize this is the first time you cry. You have always been a disappointment to them. Here you go again, producing a dead baby instead of a living one.

Someone puts a long needle in your back and tells you it will help ease the pain, but it does not.

Finally, you tell them you have decided on the C-section because she has been dead for days and you cannot get her out. You have failed many times at this whole motherhood thing: you can neither produce a living child nor deliver her properly. They wheel you down the hall. You ask them to give you a strong sedative for the surgery, and they do. But still you can see the blank faces of the doctors, the bright lights and tubes tied to your arms, and you still feel the pulling when they get her out. They seem to hand her to a nurse, who quickly leaves with a large blanket. You don't know where they have taken her.

When you are in a new room and the surgery is over, you are so happy the belly has gone that you breathe a sigh of relief. Think: "It is over!" For many years, regret this thought. You have wished for an "over," but there is no "over." Rather, there is a before and after. There is so much of a before and after that some days you can no longer stand the sight of your smiling wedding photographs, before you knew what was to be soon after. Or not be.

Your parents come to the hospital and talk briefly and seriously. They remember a friend whose baby died during her pregnancy forty years ago, who had to wait months to deliver. "Before Pitocin," they say.

"Oh," you say, "that is sad."

They place a salmon-coloured mug with an attached spoon and some white carnations on the windowsill of your room. Later, when they are gone, open the small envelope attached to it and read what they wrote: "Get well soon."

Funny, you think. You did not know you were sick.

The midwife comes in and tells you they took pictures. You are surprised at this news: surely, there was nothing to take pictures of. You cannot even imagine it. When she tells you that the baby had a beautiful face, whimper softly because when they told you she was dead, you had thought she was a monster. Try to picture the baby with a body and a face, but you cannot.

A nurse who seems flighty and overworked but not necessarily unkind reveals to you the dead child you produced was a girl, even though you have asked not to be told the sex. A daughter. This is all you have ever wanted. You were waiting all this time for that girl, that beautifully gendered baby girl.

For two days, you do not want to see her. Finally, on the third day, you say it is ok when they ask and you wait. A different nurse opens the door and comes in with a small bundle wrapped in a white crocheted blanket. Later, they will give you this blanket to take home, when it is empty. She places the bundle in your arms, and it has a tiny knit hat so all you can see is the face. The nurse tells you not to take her hat off because of the autopsy, it is resewn. Think: "Frankenstein's monster." Look carefully at her face. Think about touching the dark hair sticking out from under the hat, but you do not do it because you are afraid. Her face is perfect, with a tiny nose between some light bruises and above her bright red lips. When you touch her forehead with your finger, you are surprised it is cold. She is tiny but heavy so you give her away quickly. See, in the corner of your eye, your husband crying and kissing her face again and again. You can only kiss it once before you hand her back because it is very, very cold.

Years later, your biggest regret is this: giving her back so quickly. Now, though, it seems like enough, and you are frightened and just want to go home. List the things no one tells you about pregnancy: the swollen ankles, the difficulty breathing when you walk up stairs quickly, the questions from strangers, and you only get to take your baby home if you have produced a living one.

Also, later, when she is gone, you wish you had thought to look at her feet.

REFRAIN

At home, at first, it is better. You can take the sleeping pills they prescribed for you and sleep in your own bed, even though you cannot lie on your side from the pain and you must wear a sports bra at all times. Once, when you take it off to shower, look carefully at your nipple and see the white liquid you produced for her leaking out.

When you wake in the morning, feel fine, refreshed, the sleeping pills must help! Then: remember it. Remember it all.

Look in the mirror at what you have: a bereaved body living in two times at once. Your pregnant body was two bodies, but now you are less than one.

Later, when you are out of sleeping pills and still in bed, you cannot sleep. And you are very, very alone: there is no person in your belly and no baby on the outside. Where did she go? Oh, right: you lost her. Look quickly behind you like a woman who is losing her mind.

At night, when you try to fall asleep again, hear a baby crying. Try to shut this off. Instead, get up and look around for the baby, even in the basement. Check the washing machine. Say: "Just in case." Remember: when you were in the hospital trying to force your uterus to contract and deliver your dead baby, you heard living babies crying too.

You have a dream that you are giving birth in the hospital, pushing hard, and they place a tiny white kitten on your chest. They tell you the kitten will die. When you wake up, think: "Oh, thank god! It was only a kitten!"

Send your husband back to the hospital for the baby's things. There is a tiny handmade box with her pictures and the white blanket inside it. In the photographs, she is long, stretched out. This bothers you. In them, she is lifeless, with red lips, darkness around her eyes, and a bruised body. You can see how she should have been moving. Seven pounds, three ounces. Say: "Perfect." Touch the picture of her face and put it away.

The next day, look through what you have left: a couple of photographs, some black footprints, a small teddy bear the nurse placed between her hands in the pictures, a pink hat, and a cast of your big belly you took on one of the last days.

The baby room door is closed. Behind the door, there is a lamp in the shape of a rabbit. There is a hand-me-down crib, a dresser, and a sketch of a bunny and a dragonfly you bought and framed.

When the midwife comes later, beg her for specifics because you cannot remember. Do you remember the doctor putting a probe into you to find out if you were contracting during those days you spent trying to get her out? "No," you say, you do not remember. You do remember the midwife rubbing your feet. You remember asking her if you would have to push. You remember when she told you your milk would come in, you covered your chest with one arm and sobbed. When you were pregnant with a living baby, this was the only way you could imagine her: nursing at your breast, a tiny hand in your hand, a sweet smelling head on your chest.

Ask the midwife about that smell. The lock of hair they taped to her footprints smells like a baby. Say: "What is that? I always thought it was baby powder."

"No," she says and shakes her head, "babies smell sweet." This makes the tears run down your face without stopping, thinking about the sweet smell of babies. Your baby.

Get up and check the mailbox. For ten days in a row, you get one sympathy card or more in the mail before they end, and you don't need to check the mail anymore. Your mother's sister writes in her card that her cat Gizzy died. Crumble the card and throw it into the trash.

When spring comes, try to go for a walk. See the overabundance of mothers with living babies walking them in strollers. Then, getting on the school bus, there are little girls. They have pretty dresses and barrettes in their hair. Soon you cannot even go to the corner pharmacy. Try the supermarket instead. When you are in a long line behind a mother and a small baby, abandon a cart full of groceries and walk quickly to your car in the parking lot.

Tell yourself you will one day again cook dinner or play the piano, but today is not that day. You cannot read or listen to music: these are the things you and she used to do together.

Go to the baby store to buy a baby book during your one moment of hope that someday there will be a living baby in your house. On the shelf, you see a machine to listen to your baby's heartbeat. Pick it up and read the outside of the box, the long paragraph describing how it can be used to prevent stillbirth. It ends with an exclamation point. Place your chin to your chest. Why, why did you not get that machine?

On a good day, you feel like it will be ok, that someday you will be a mother. On a bad day, it is not even close.

Imagine yourself dead. Imagine yourself pregnant. Decide you want both, or perhaps neither. Think hard about how you will answer the question, "How many children do you have?"

Keep a list of things people should and should not say to a mom like you. Under "OK" write: "We miss her too" and "I'm so sorry." Under "Not OK" write: "I can't believe you missed my birthday" and "You are not the same person." These are the most painful ones—written in the letters you get later on from the people who were supposed to be your friends. One of the worst ones ends with "This is not the you I know." Remember: you no longer know yourself.

Shut up, you say to the letter. Shut shut shut up. Soon phone calls from these people make you throw up violently and without warning like you did when you were first pregnant. Unplug the phone.

Think about death. Wish for your own, wish to go back to the moment of hers. You were there, after all, watching her slip quietly away.

List things that are difficult: peeing next to the baby changer attached to the wall in the department store bathroom. Ordering coffee next to the woman in line fussing over a baby picture. Walking by the baby clothes in the superstore. Tiny shoes of any colour. "Mommy!" called by a small child.

Try not to wince when people show off their pregnant bellies.

Years later, still notice the gap: the family portraits, the number of grandchildren, the order of the cousins, the preschool class, the bus for school children passing your house, the father daughter party no one has invited your husband to attend. This will continue for years to come but now, you do not yet know this, and it is somehow better.

Keep your list of "OK" and "Not OK" in case you need to add to it later, which of course you do.

SUSTAINED

There is a support group for people like you. When you go, you hear the term "babyloss mama" for the first time. Think: you do not want to be here. You do not want to be one of them. Baby loss mama. The word mama is there but with some horrible identifier in front of it.

"I always feel like some kind of dead baby mama freak bag," says one. Say: "Oh, you too?"

Another one says, "When I held her in the hospital, I cried and cried all over her because I wanted my tears to go with her when they took her away."

"Oh," you say, "that was a good idea." Curse yourself for not thinking of that. The one with the unwashed hair says, "When people ask me why she died, I don't know what to say because probably I killed her."

"How did you think you killed her?" you ask. She gulps and coughs and wipes the tears off her cheek. She says, "I drank a cup of coffee and that was probably it." You try not to laugh. This is ridiculous. This is trying to get the maternal body to behave responsibly. Coffee is at fault for none of this.

After the meeting, think: you yourself almost certainly killed your baby by not paying enough attention. Or maybe it was that soft cheese. Another miscalculating mother at fault.

You start seeing a therapist. She starts many sentences with "other parents who have lost children tell me," but often you cannot make out the rest because you sob loudly. You are glad for this phrasing, though, especially the "other parents" part. You don't know them, but you imagine them in their big suburban houses with their other children running in the yard. Funny, they are dead baby freak bags too.

Your husband, who is both an atheist and a physicist, takes you to where they have put her ashes. It is behind a big gate and full of plants and trees. He insists her molecules are with us. He can calculate this. "See," he says, scratching some numbers on a wrinkled yellow page from a legal pad, "there she is." He grins proudly and circles the dots on the page.

Later, when you are alone, throw some dirt in the air. Watch it fall down, get into your hair, and leave dust on your face. Whisper: "I miss you." Say it out loud: "I miss you, baby girl."

12.
How to Hear a Story

Reflections on the Anniversary of My Rape

RHOBI JACOBS

The truth about stories is that's all we are.
—Thomas King

I AM A STORYTELLER. It's what I do for a living, I mean.
In my early twenties, I was paid to tell the tales of families. My job was to tell the stories of their problems: the bills spewing out of the mailbox; the daycares that fell through; the jobs that changed often; how someone's kid ran away again; how someone shaved every inch of hair to avoid failing another drug test. I trailed behind them with a clipboard. I took notes about the details so that I could write up their stories later in the office while I slurped coffee from a ceramic mug shaped like a crumpled cardboard cup. I was writing these stories to present, ultimately, to a judge, somewhere in the jurisdiction, who would use my stories to assign merit to a family. The way I told these stories, and the details contained within, shaped the fate of every family I encountered.

When I tired of that, I moved to hospital stories: stories of people who had to come to live on the quarantine ward for complicated tuberculosis. My notes were shorter for these stories because everyone else was writing them too—the nurses and the doctors and all the people hired to play chess and do yoga with these devastated in-patients. Us attendants told their stories to each other, and we wrote these stories in the lined papers that would later fill the cabinets in a basement room under the rehab wing. These stories were caught and tacked like dead moths to inspect. There was no life in them—certainly I didn't live in them, and the patients didn't live in them, either. They were factual, coded. Even where they had detailed the warm aspects of a life—the nuances of a feeling, a longing for death or freedom, or a request to be moved to a room with a garden view—these live elements were shaken off from them, and the leftovers flattened for efficiency and stored away for an infinity.

I'm done with that now, though.

Now, I tell stories of my own. My own stories are live and lithe, and as slippery as fish. They resist lying flat between the lines of paper.

I'll tell you one, if you like.

First, you should know it didn't happen in January. People care about the facts when you tell them this kind of story, so you'd better get them right. And we were living in the city, but that's not where it happened. It happened in summertime, in my smallish hometown, where you don't get a doctor's note for having a dead baby.

The ultrasound lady was named Gail or Gwen or Greer or—on second thought, maybe it was something else. We were at a walk-in place offering 3D images; it had a wall-mounted screen on which to watch, and that's how I knew before she told me so that my baby was already dead. Seeing him there, all curled up and still—he was beautiful, my second son.

The woman was empathic. She gazed at me with tears in her eyes before calling the radiologist, who led us to her office, where she dialed the midwife's receptionist, who summoned the midwife, who had to tell us over one of those square black-and-grey office phones from 1992.

The midwife's voice was small as she told me that our baby had died weeks earlier but my body had plunged along still pregnant and unaware. She told me that I was only going into labour now and that I'd have to go to the ER without her. Actually, she didn't use the word labour. In fact, she didn't explain anything at all.

* * *

The day after my rape, I drove deep into the country with my husband. I rested my wilted head on the gape of the open window and let the whipping air pound into me, into my eyes and sobbing mouth, into my ears and nose. My sound was a strange animal as I watched the fields flick endlessly by, their tall grass bending to me, the loam below opening to me as if my grave. I could not die, and I was not dead. Neither was I a living thing, animated with spirit, nor was I fully functioning. It was as if my spirit had emptied from its corporeal case, and I was not soul or flesh.

I am going to tell you about the corporality of memory—how we take experiences of particular pleasure or trauma into our cells, how deeply we bank them, how they transform from physical experience into the stuff of our dreams, our poems and songs, our beliefs about ourselves and our agency and our futures. These are the ways our stories of loss and transgression exist beyond and apart from the evidentiary dimension of rape or the medical event of miscarriage. This is a recollection about both.

In *The Body Remembers Casebook*, a guide to treatment methods for post-traumatic stress disorder (PTSD) and trauma, Babette Rothschild describes the ways our memories store information:

> There are basically two major types of memory: implicit and explicit. Explicit memory is conscious and requires language. It comprises concepts, facts, events, descriptions, and thoughts. Implicit memory, on the other hand, is unconscious. It is made up of emotions, sensations, movements, and automatic procedures. The terms "body memory" and "somatic memory" suggest the implicit. (8)

An internationally renowned psychotherapist and social worker specializing in PTSD, Rothschild makes this important distinction between types of memory to outline the complexity of how we carry trauma in our physical selves, not just our minds. She explains as follows:

> Body sensations that constitute emotions (e.g., terror) and physical states (e.g. pain or [Autonomic Nervous System] arousal), and the patterns that make up movements (e.g., fight, flight, freeze) are all recorded in the brain. Sometimes the corresponding explicit elements—e.g. the facts of the

situation, a description of the events—are simultaneously recorded; sometimes they are not. (10)

In this description, we can begin to understand how a storyteller's "physical" memories of an event (that is, how the instinctual brain instructs the body to experience the trauma) may be misaligned with the details of the event. It is even possible, according to Rothschild and others, that a survivor may miss the facts of a situation entirely. It is more than reasonable for a storyteller of this kind to rely on other markers of the experience (feelings, emotions, sensations) or what I call "soft markers"—fluid understandings of time, place, context—in their understanding of and subsequent retelling of a traumatic event. Similarly, people who have survived trauma may say they were outside their body, because of the dual selves at work: one keeps watch (or forgets to), while the other moves through the event as it is taking place. We are not just our material selves; we are not just the particles making up the mass of us. We are also the metaphysical experience of being a live thing. We are complex and delicate.

* * *

What is it like to be raped? My sisters and I will tell you: we feel we are etherized with experience and intensity. We are beside ourselves. Then, we are souls driven out of flesh—our stellar orbital selves still intact—although our bodies lie down. In time, maybe: the stitching of soul to skin, the cautious, tender remerging of self, a careful grafting. Looking toward or looking away, how the story haunts us. It is long before we ascend our own incredulity. It is eternal sometimes.

We are a subtle sisterhood, those of us who have been transgressed, and we grapple with the truth of our narrative. We want the experience to include the story of our harm. We want the story of our harm to include the meaning of our experience—to carry with it the many days it takes to decide to relive or to ignore the shock, the bewilderment of being so wholly, intentionally wronged in the time of deepest vulnerability. All the while our bodies assert their own truth, spontaneously delivering messages of absent danger.

* * *

On 19 June 2010, I went into the local hospital in labour with my second son, whose death had been confirmed earlier that day via 4D ultrasound. The technician hadn't meant to show us in 4D; she forgot to change the output of her screen. But there he was on the wall-mounted plasma TV like a tiny piece of carved moon rock.

I had gone into labour in the park where the local mothers gather every day in the heat of high summer. The big kids played in the muck, and the adults and little ones sprawled on a blanket and talked about the birds and the bees. I'd been feeling strange all morning but chalked it up to the heat until a warm bomb of liquid slipped out between my legs. I hurried to the outhouse, anxious and embarrassed, and found blood there, deep red and smelling of iron.

The day after my labour, I drove to the country with my husband. We drove with the window open, the threads of the baby quilt I'd been making streamed out into the air. We drove further and further, and I was a rattling cicada, sounding loud, trembling and ancient. When we stopped, I said nothing. I plucked a leaf of wild sage or castilleja or dandelion, and, gathering some loose yellow threads from my quilt, tied it tight to the big door of an empty church.

* * *

In her paper "Less Pain, More Gain," psychotherapist Angel Yuen wonders, "what can be made possible when we are actively curious about how a person has responded to trauma, rather than only focusing on how they were affected by it?" (7). This distinction between the internalized matter of an event and the chronological unfolding of an event is subtle but important to survivors of assault, and it is in keeping with the concepts of implicit and explicit memory that Rothschild talks about. Chronology is the luxury of the conscious mind, and trauma does not reside there. Chronology and the associated details of action (who was where, and how, and when) are elements of the story, but they are not the truth of the story. Although they may compile a formal disclosure, they are not essentially the useful parts. Not to me, anyway.

You have heard me say that I am strong—or, you have heard me say that I was wronged. And you are looking, probably, for the details. You are probably looking for the details so that you can know whose fault it was. Or, at least, how it happened. Or maybe you want the details so that you can know how to respond to me, or to someone, or to my sister. You want from me. You want from my story.

It's okay. I offered. Kind of.

* * *

David Epston and Michael White say that "narrative therapy ... situates an individual at the center of her or his therapeutic journey and acknowledges the individual as 'the expert in their own life'" (4). Thus, my storytelling is part of the process of extricating the problem from my internal being. I am trying to lend time to undertaking what Epston and White call the process of "storying and restorying" the event, while my external context shifts, and the poignant elements of the trauma surface. My telling is also rooted in the desire for my listener to understand how I move about in the world—carrying out the work of mothering, storytelling, healing, and helping—in the context of my survival of trauma.

You should know, though, that this need to tell is often problematic, even as it can serve in my healing. As I narrate, my goal is to highlight those elements of the story that are themes of my personal strength and resilience. But at the same time, the potential for a listener whose interest is about the details—and not, as Yeun has mentioned, my *response* to the details—poses a risk to the integrity and usefulness of my sharing.

I mean that it is not useful, on the whole, for the listener to hear my story—unless that listener has also endured some similar trauma and has lived, as some people have lived, long in secret silence wondering at the words for it. In this instance (I would say this is the single instance of helpfulness), my telling is about the listener as much as it is about my story. But a strange and separate thing often happens when I share that I was raped during my miscarriage: my listener takes on a role of co-perpetrator in their expectation I provide the details of my experience. It's not intentional, but the dynamic exists just the same: I must prove my story, I must prove myself, I must prove my passive role in the trauma.

This feeling of having to offer proof is characteristic of many people who survive abuse. It's a phenomenon we are becoming especially familiar with in light of social commentary on rape culture. It's about a listener just wanting the details, just wanting those stories to somehow make more sense. But it, at best, communicates mostly innocuous disbelief, and, at worst, it represents a deeply rooted sexism. To expect a disclosure is to ally with the perpetrator instead of the survivor.

This is an uncomfortable truth. For most everyone, the goal of asking questions in response to a story of trauma is certainly not to cause more grief or to reintroduce anguish. Probably there isn't any goal at all. Rather, we aren't sure how to receive a story that fails to contextualize an event, and in our uncertainty about our ability to hear and make sense of it, we react. We want details where we should sit with our sense of disorientation because that reflects the experience of assault and loss we are hearing. It is no failure of the storyteller if a listener can't get her bearings; it's just the nature of this type of narrative. The facts are hard to know, and hard to speak, and hard to hear—but the good news is that they aren't precursors to understanding a story because this type of story is about how a happening settled in and what that means now.

A truly allied listener can attend to the story without evaluating what a storyteller has included or omitted from her description of an event. For one thing, part of the difficulty of restorying a pregnancy loss for the individual at its centre is that as an event, it is a-chronological. Babies are not supposed to die before they are birthed. Parents are not supposed to bury or mourn what they have not yet welcomed. And still, in our integration of these stories, the chronology of a thing is important. As an expectant parent, your baby's life is tracked in weeks and days, and your own body's changes follow suit. Later, you may know the time of death because of the smallness of your baby, even it takes weeks more to birth the body.

Although time and place may be part of a narrative of loss or trauma, they are not the central plot. When we force the formulation of a fact-based assimilative timeline through question asking, instead of receiving a narrative as a listener void of expectation (that the story have a complete timeline or congruent plot, for example), we cannot actively receive the nuanced details. We risk discrediting the voice of the teller. When we get caught up in specificity as listeners, we communicate that the extraneous details hold more worth than the intrinsic meaning a survivor has assigned to her story.

And anyway, the story doesn't stay the same. Not because I intend to change it, not because mine is an unreliable account (although it may be), but because the story is as alive as I am alive.

What I mean is all stories morph. It is necessary for the personal narrative to subsume the details of (formal) disclosure to rise above the chaos of the experience and respond to the event first in a physical and very literal way and, later, in spiritual and emotional acts of meaning-making. Crisis gives way to shifts in identity, whereas narrative and our own telling of the story is about the pursuit of justice, even though we might never make a formal disclosure. Justice happens when I get to decide what this story means for and about me; justice is being in control of how and to whom I present the details; it's about how I come to know myself through them.

When we allow for the fragmented, fluid stories of rape and loss to come out, and when we receive these stories well—alive and disorienting as they are—we are constructing a way of knowing that values the whole truth of a thing and places the person at the centre of their narrative. This is critical to the development of a feminist epistemology of trauma and loss because of the way it recentralizes an individual in the process of meaning-making. It is congruent with feminist concepts of reproductive justice: in essence, it says, "my story, my choice."

So, I want to give you the story with searing edges. I want to give it to you because I know that there is poetry in my powerlessness, my womanhood, my sisterhood, my words. I have chosen to give these things to you and I am redeemed in them, regardless of the details. Because the story changes consistency as I grow. It stretches, in places, it bends. It is in me and it is me and it is mine to tell.

WORKS CITED

Epston, David, and Michael White. *Experience, Contradiction, Narrative & Imagination: Selected Papers of David Epston & Michael White, 1989-1991.* Dulwich Centre Publications, 1992.

King, Thomas. *The Truth about Stories: A Native Narrative.* University of Minnesota, 2005.

Rothschild, Babette. *The Body Remembers Casebook: Unifying Methods and Models in the Treatment of Trauma* and PTSD. New Norton & Company, Inc., 2003.

Yuen, Angel. "Less Pain, More Gain: Explorations of Response versus Effects When Working with the Consequences of Trauma." *Explorations: An E-journal of Narrative Practice*, vol. 1, no. 1, 2009, pp. 6-16.

IV. INTERROGATING THE MEDICALIZED LOGICS OF PREGNANCY LOSS

13.
A Death Certificate, an Autopsy Report, a Pile of Insurance Claims

ELIZABETH HEINEMAN

I AM THE homebirthing community's worst nightmare. I am the one who had a stillbirth—a stillbirth that probably would not have occurred had I been receiving hospital care.

My midwife made a judgment call. Doctors make judgment calls too. But when their judgment calls turn out to be wrong, it doesn't call into question the entire enterprise of hospital birth.

When their judgment calls turn out to be wrong, no one blames the mother for having chosen hospital birth.

At my last prenatal checkup, at forty-one-weeks-two-days, my nurse-midwife did not recommend induction. She did not recommend an ultrasound. An ultrasound probably would not tell us anything we didn't already know, she said. And what we already knew was this: my pregnancy was uncomplicated, my blood pressure low, my fetal nonstress tests good, my amniotic fluid plentiful, and my cervix two centimetres dilated and 80 percent effaced. I was of advanced maternal age, neither overweight nor underweight; I was fit, not a smoker, not a drinker, not a drug user. I did not have gestational diabetes. I did not have preeclampsia. My first baby had been postdate too. Simple vaginal delivery.

The hospital would have ordered an ultrasound anyway because it had a schedule, and the schedule said: forty-weeks-five-days means time for an ultrasound. The hospital would have induced anyway because it had a schedule, and the schedule said: forty-one weeks means time to induce. Even if induction means increased likelihood of further intervention for a pregnancy showing no sign of trouble, for a pregnancy that may not be postdate at all, since you don't always know exactly when you got pregnant. Those due dates are just estimates.

My midwife said: at your next prenatal visit, in two days, we will revisit the possibility of an ultrasound. If there *is* a next prenatal visit, she joked.

There wasn't. When I went into labour the next evening, my midwife came by. She heard the baby's strong heartbeat, noted the bloody show, and saw I was still only two centimetres dilated and 80 percent effaced. We should call her when my contractions reached sixty seconds or my water broke. She lived two blocks away and would be back in five minutes once we called.

And so we were alone, as we would have been had I gone into labour naturally while planning a hospital birth. The hospital doesn't want you coming in when your contractions are mild and twenty-five-seconds long, and you are walking around, eating toast and reading comics to pass the time. It will be a while yet, and there's no need for you to take a bed for twelve or twenty-four hours, a bed that might be needed by someone who's closer to delivery.

But I was forty-one-weeks-three-days. If I had been planning a hospital delivery, I would have been induced. And if I had been induced, I would have been in the hospital from the beginning, and so I would have been in the hospital when the short, mild contractions turned ferocious barely an hour later and a few drops of bright red blood trickled down my leg. It would not have been up to me and my partner to interpret the blood, to interpret contractions that cut like a knife and came quickly but were still only forty-seconds long. Second deliveries often go faster than first deliveries, right? Birth involves blood, right? Whether or not the doctors would have discovered that my placenta had, all at once, separated from my uterus, they would have known something was wrong, and they would have intervened.

Or perhaps the placental abruption would not have occurred at all. Perhaps with induced labour starting a day or two earlier than natural labour did, my placenta would have stayed where it belonged on the uterine wall, until the baby was born. And then it would have slipped easily out, like an exhalation, just like it did for my first baby, and I would have planted it under a tree, which we would visit years later to see how it had grown.

When my midwife arrived—five minutes after we called, like she promised—there was no heartbeat. My cervix had gone from two to eight centimetres in two hours. My body was trying to get the baby out fast because the baby was in trouble. It was too late for a hospital transfer. The midwife burst the amniotic sac to hurry things along, and dark brown meconium poured out, chunky, like diarrhea.

* * *

I spent my pregnancy furious at the American medical system. I was furious at it for making a nearly one-third chance of a C-section the price I would have to pay for the fastest possible access to emergency care if it should be necessary. I should not have been faced with that choice.

I knew that the World Health Organization estimates the optimal C-section rate to be no more than 15 percent. If the American C-section rate is 30 percent—humour me here, I know that number is a little low, but only a little, and it keeps the numbers nice and round—then submitting yourself to that system brings a 15 percent risk of unnecessary C-section. The rate of placental abruption is between one half and 1 percent. That includes women with major risk factors like smoking, cocaine use, and high blood pressure. But let's say my risk of a placental abruption was 1 percent. My risk of unnecessary C-section in the hospital would have been at least fifteen times higher.

At least your baby would have lived through an unnecessary C-section.

You're right. My baby would have lived.

Though let's be consistent. If we're going to think "worst-case scenario" about homebirth, we may as well think "worst-case scenario" about hospital birth too. "Worst-case scenario" does not mean unnecessary C-section. "Worst-case scenario" means the doctor's judgment call is in keeping with the standard of care but turns out to be fatal, as it was for my friend's sister. "Worst-case scenario" means your unnecessary C-section turns into one of the nearly hundred thousand unnecessary deaths in hospitals each year—deaths due to infection introduced by a technician who washes his hands improperly, or an overtired resident who misplaces a decimal point when scribbling her order for medication, or a doctor who is too proud to hear an underling's warnings that there's something wrong.

Or is it forty thousand deaths? A hundred ninety-five thousand? I don't know; it depends on which study you read, and I'm too sick of this whole mess to sort it out.

No, I don't think any of those things would have happened to me if I'd planned a hospital birth. The odds are vastly against their happening to any one person.

And so someone else becomes the statistic for unnecessary stillbirth in the hospital while I become the statistic for unnecessary stillbirth at home.

* * *

What remains is the inventory of my son's life:

A death certificate, an autopsy report, a pile of insurance claims.

Photos of him, dull eyes half open, here in his father's arms, here in mine.

A funeral program with verses by Goethe and Toni Morrison.

Drops of milk that I squeeze from my nipples, fifteen months later, so I can watch the water from the showerhead dilute them into invisibility before washing them down the drain.

* * *

Author's note: My stillbirth was in November 2008, but I have spoken and written about it many times since. To portray my experience and decision-making honestly, I must step back in time to 2008, to the data then available, and to the discussions in the media at that time. This piece—originally written in 2010—reflects that effort. Since 2008, new studies and media representations have changed the discussion for some medical professionals and expectant mothers as well as the larger public. A major study of homebirths was released in 2014, for example, and was promptly interpreted as either endorsing or damning homebirth, depending on the position of the commentator (Cheyney et al.). In 2017, the American College of Obstetrics and Gynecology endorsed a report outlining recommendations to limit interventions during normal labour and delivery. I have not updated this piece to reference recent research, however, since it expresses my interpretation of my experience at the time.

Because of the literary nature of this piece, I choose not to break it up with citations. Below you will find citations of the data available to me in 2008, although in this works cited list, some of those data are embedded in more recent reports. The citations below were not necessarily my sources at the time (I did not keep careful records), but they convey the same information.

This chapter was previously published in Hip Mama Magazine, *number 47, 2010.*

WORKS CITED

Cheyney, Melissa, et al. "Outcomes of Care for 16,924 Planned Home Births in the United States: The Midwives Alliance of North America Statistics Project, 2004 to 2009." *Journal of Midwifery and Women's Health*, vol. 59, no. 1, 2014, pp. 17-27.

"Infections due to Hand-Washing Failures Cause 100,000 Deaths Annually," *News Medical Life Sciences*, 17 Sept. 2009, www.news-medical.net/news/20090917/Infections-due-to-handwashing-failures-cause-100000-deaths-annually.aspx. Accessed 13 Sept. 2017.

"In Hospital Deaths from Medical Errors at 195,000 per Year in USA." *Medical News Today*, 9 Aug. 2004, www.medicalnewstoday.com/releases/11856.php. Accessed 13 Sept. 2017.

Menacker, Fay, and Brady E. Hamilton. "Recent Trends in Cesarean Delivery in the United States." *Centers for Disease Control and Prevention*, March 2010, www.cdc.gov/nchs/data/databriefs/db35.pdf. Accessed 13 Sept. 2017.

Shad H. Deering et al. "Abruptio Placentae." *Medscape*, 23 Nov. 2016, emedicine.medscape.com/article/252810-overview. Accessed 13 Sept. 2017.

The American College of Obstetricians and Gynecologists Committee Opinion. "Approaches to Limit Intervention during Labor and Birth." *ACOG*, Feb. 2017, *www.acog.org/Resources-And-Publi-*

cations/Committee-Opinions/Committee-on-Obstetric-Practice/
Approaches-to-Limit-Intervention-During-Labor-and-Birth.
Accessed 13 Sept. 2017.

World Health Organization. "Statement on Caesarian Section Rates."
WHO, 2015, apps.who.int/iris/bitstream/10665/161442/1/
WHO_RHR_15.02_eng.pdf. Accessed 13 Sept. 2017.

14.
Failing Fertility

A Case to Queer the Rhetoric of Infertility

MARIA NOVOTNY

It is amazing how much silence surrounds the struggle of infertility. The silence of not wanting to talk about it. The silence of wanting to talk about it, but being scared. The silence of trying to avoid the one thing you are wondering about, but not wanting to focus on it, and yet having your mind dominated by it. The silence of not feeling comfortable talking with others about it because it involves sex. The silence because you just don't want to deal with the questions. That silence gives shame all the voice it needs to whisper silently, 'Something is wrong with you.' Infertility is a shame-filled, silent trial, isolating couples in closed bedrooms of pain.—Nate Pyle, *The Huffington Post*

You have to grieve the loss of your fertility because it is such an integral part of being a woman.—Amanda Aldrich (qtd. in Barhite)

TO UNDERSTAND INFERTILITY as a heteronormative cisgender woman is to understand it as a deeply disorienting experience in which women live in a state of wanting to be but are not yet pregnant (Sandelowski; Tjornhog-Thomsen). Although young women in America are frequently taught in sexual education classes and public health campaigns to take precautions with their sexual activity, the rhetoric behind such messaging suggests cautioning female sexuality because of a presumptive need to safeguard female fertility. Female sexuality in this context correlates to female fertility and hence, unwanted pregnancy. As such, young girls are taught from the beginning they are fertile beings and need to protect themselves against an unwanted pregnancy to ensure a future filled with opportunities for success. Yet, as these young girls mature into young adult women, the messaging shifts. No longer must young adult women protect their fertility; instead, they now must be proactive about their fertility. Adult women must be "smart" and "plan" for not only *how* they will support their children but *when* they should start thinking about having children. The metaphorical "ticking clock" emerges.

Still, little sexual education messaging—whether in regards to young girls or mature women—focuses upon the reality that becoming pregnant is not necessarily an easy feat. Thus, when a woman in her early thirties makes the shift to no longer protect her fertility and, instead, chooses to become pregnant but encounters difficulty, feelings of frustration, anger, and sadness emerge. The messages she was told from an early age no longer seem true. As a result, coming to terms with an infertile identity, particularly as a self-identified female, is a grief-filled and disorienting process affecting identity formation and feelings of self-worthlessness. Research aimed to better understand women's emotional grief frequently accompanying their infertility diagnosis explains: "During childhood and adolescence, social messages about the importance of parenthood are constantly disseminated and especially for women, being a mother is something often central to identity. Thus, a sense of loss of identity and feelings of defectiveness and incompetence are quite often experienced" (Galhardo et al. 2409).

Women are continually taught that their fertility already is, can and must be controlled so as to fulfill these cultural expectations of female identity. Yet when women learn they cannot control their fertility by experiencing infertility, internalized shame takes root. Infertility demands grieving not only the inability to naturally conceive a child but also the cultural and normative notions of being a woman: "From the vantage point of American infertile women ... infertility is a major disruption in one's projected life course, a failure to live up to normative notions about what it means to be an adult woman in American society, and a challenge to the stability and quality of social relationships" (Greil 101).

In Western culture, the fertile female then is viewed as normed and desired. Unable to live up to these cultural expectations, many infertile women silently experience feelings of deep shame, which give root to the stigmatization of infertility (Slauson-Blevins et al.). Linda Whiteford and Lois Gonzalez write, "for many infertile women in North America infertility is a secret stigma, distinguished from more obvious examples of stigmatization because it is invisible" (28). The invisibility of infertility leaves many infertile individuals further marginalized because Western cultural norms are oriented around family ideals. Everyday interactions can become harder and more difficult for infertile individuals, particularly women, to encounter. From the Facebook post of a friend's child at the zoo, to the pregnant woman buying groceries, and to the even more mundane reused diaper box a neighbour drops off with some perennials—all can trigger feelings of deep frustration and sadness, and leave many infertile individuals wondering, will I ever share in such an experience?

Infertility's invisibility, as well as Western culture's presumed association of fertility with femininity, can make the decision to disclose one's infertility a difficult and even risky choice. Wanting to protect their privacy, many infertile women silently hide their infertility diagnosis. Yet studies have noted how silence often perpetuates and protects the stigma of infertility, as it "sustains the myth of fertility as a universal experience, suppressing contrary experiences in an ideology of motherhood and symbolic ideal of family" (Allison 17).

Drawing on the role of silence as a rhetorical mechanism to maintain normative Western cultural conceptions of fertility, this chapter examines the intersections between shame, stigma and reproductive grief. By highlighting how contemporary discourses of infertility are currently situated within Western medicine, I demonstrate how rhetorics of shame enhance the stigmatization of infertility and act as a systemic-like sister to the medical discourse of infertility. Specifically, I posit that infertility operates akin to the Althusserian construct of "always, already." For Louis Althusser, discourse mediates ideology in which language naturalizes as a function. Discourse is always and already presumed to be supportive of a particular ideological position. Applying an

Althusserian approach to infertility as discourse, reveals how the medicalized discourse of infertility reinforces normative ideologies of the female body as a fertile body. What results is a medicalized discursive ideology dictating that to be an infertile female is to live in an abnormal body.

This medical discourse becomes reinforced through biomedical technological practices that controls and reaffirms the construction of a normal female body as a fertile female body, whereas an abnormal female body is an infertile female body. An example of biomedical practices reaffirming such ideological constructions is the use of, and general cultural acceptance toward, reproductive technologies, such as in vitro fertilization (IVF). Fertility clinics and Western culture's turn to IVF as a solution to "conquering" or "beating" infertility fails to account for larger ideological underpinnings affecting constructions of gender, sexuality and the family. Mamo in *Mommy Queerest* echoes a similar position on the effects of biomedicalization on the infertile body" "discourses of (medical) reproduction and sexuality co-produce subjectivities and social forms of biomedical belonging" (10). Although biomedical practices such as IVF may resolve some infertile women's desire to have a family, I argue these medicalized discourses and practices actually reinforce a stigmatization about infertility, particularly in the context of gender and sexuality—that is to be infertile, especially as a woman, is to be perceived as less female. My objective in pointing to such deficit discourses accompanying female infertility is to draw parallels between infertility and discussions of non-normativity that frequently appear in queer theory. To support this claim, I provide a brief case study of an infertility organization that attempts to advocate on behalf of infertile women and men. It demonstrates that although their advocacy efforts attempt to usurp stigmas of infertility, their activist rhetoric and strategies reinforce the medicalization of infertility. Ultimately, I posit the organization fails to achieve its mission to reduce the stigma of infertility. To better support their mission and advocacy efforts, I turn to queer theory as a source that not only shares in experiences of stigmatization, shame, and non-normativity, but may provide more critical insight into challenging the systemic and deficit-filled labelling of infertility. Queering the rhetoric of infertility, I believe, may queer infertile women's perceptions of their infertile bodies, challenging discourses that systemically label the infertile female body as non-normative or deficient. Furthermore, queering the rhetoric of infertility may push the infertile community to embrace and develop more critical activist rhetorics that resist dominant discourses of infertility.

THE MEDICALIZATION OF INFERTILITY

Over the years, infertility has evolved into an ambiguous medical condition. Definitions vary regarding how infertility is assessed and measured (Gurunath et. al). Nonetheless, most researchers agree that contemporary understandings should view infertility "as a socially constructed process whereby individuals come to regard their inability to have children as a problem, to define the nature of that problem, and to construct an appropriate course of action" (Greil et al. 737). Frequently, this course of action directs infertile couples to seek medical treatment. Today, one in eight couples experience infertility, and approximately 85 to 90 percent of these infertility cases are being treated with drug therapy or surgical procedures ("Fast Facts about Infertility"). In 2012, the Society for Assisted Reproductive Technology's annual report dictated that 165,172 assisted reproductive technology (ART) treatments, including in vitro fertilization, occurred in the United States resulting in 61,740 births (Christensen).

However, reproductive technologies that control, monitor, and make more efficient female fertility are constructed by larger societal and cultural ideologies about bodies. Michel Foucault's concept of biopower—a regulatory system that "achieves the subjugation of bodies" (140) for control—serves as frame for explaining how female fertility cultural norms are articulated through authoritative systems of knowledge, such as biomedicine. How individuals view their bodies is actually highly mediated through disciplinary systems of power, and their discourses, in the field of medicine. In this way, the medicalized language describing infertility as a disease, instead of as a socially constructed desire, discursively suggests to infertile women that their inability to conceive is because of their own bodily deficiencies. In fact, what appears when examining bodies within Foucault's biopower frame is that "bodies and their subjectivities and identifications are constituted in and through relations of power-knowledge. The classifications of 'infertility' and 'homosexuality,' for example, do not arise in nature, but are constituted by social and cultural systems of meaning, codified in cultural rules that define what is normal and abnormal" (Mamo 9).

This medicalized language embedded in discussions of infertility results in a cultural labelling of the infertile female body as non-normative and in need of medical intervention so as to resolve their infertile (and thus abnormal) female body. Such dependence on medicine to resolve infertility has constructed a rhetoric of infertility, which places value in changing the infertile body into a fertile body and in creating a discursive system devaluing the decision to accept and not fix an infertile body. This, I argue, is how deficit attitudes become entrenched in rhetorics of infertility. Specifically, these deficit attitudes reinforce feelings of shame and the stigmatization of infertility. Further evidence of this can be seen in a case study of infertility activist rhetoric.

A CASE STUDY OF RESOLVE'S[1] ADVOCACY DAY

The influential and systemic dominance of the medical rhetoric of infertility can continue to be traced to sites outside of medicine. One such example is infertility activist rhetoric. To highlight the systemic influence of the medicalization and perpetuation of deficit notions of infertility, I provide a case study Advocacy Day, a lobbying event hosted by RESOLVE, The National Infertility Association in America.

Advocacy Day is an annual event hosted by RESOLVE encouraging infertile individuals to travel to Washington D.C. and share their experiences of infertility with members of Congress. The goals of Advocacy Day are two-fold: to raise public awareness about the effects of infertility; and to make a case to Congress that infertility must be recognized legislatively as a medical disease so as to mandate national insurance coverage for fertility treatment. It is hoped that the results of Advocacy Day will affect House and Senate resolutions supporting family-building legislation

Each Advocacy Day attendee, thus, meets and advocates for

their local representative to co-sponsor three bills, preselected by RESOLVE:

The Family Act (S 881/HR 1851), which would provide eligible Americans with a tax credit for their out-of-pocket expenses incurred during IVF treatment;

The Women Veterans and Other Healthcare Improvements Act (S 131/HR 958), which would provide veterans wounded in the line of duty with access to reproductive technologies and adoption assistance;

and The Adoption Tax Credit Refundability Act of 2013 (S 1056 / HR 2144), which would increase access to the credit for low to moderate income families will make more adoptions possible for waiting children.[2]

During the morning of Advocacy Day, attendees receive their schedule for the day and are trained on how to proceed with each meeting. Specifically, attendees are encouraged to share their own personal struggle with infertility. They provide sample narratives as models for attendees. Below is a model narrative shared at the 2014 event:

> When I was in my late twenties, I was diagnosed with unexplained infertility. With treatment, I could conceive but I could never carry to term and I suffered many devastating losses. After surgery and six IVF cycles on my own, we did a 7th with a gestational surrogate with success. We had no insurance coverage for infertility and paid everything out of pocket—$58,000 in all. If The Family Act had been in place, it would have helped us make our decisions based on the most appropriate treatment instead of based on what we could afford and thereby avoid so much heartache. (*Telling Your Story*)

These narratives and preselected bills indicate RESOLVE's commitment to using medical discourses of infertility to make a case for nationally mandated insurance treatment. Specifically, RESOLVE's activist rhetoric and strategy suggest infertility is a medical disease, and, as such, it demands to be treated and resolved through fertility treatments covered via insurance. In fact, RESOLVE's rhetoric suggests the only option for infertile women to recover from their pain is through medical intervention. Furthermore, through this rhetoric, Advocacy Day reinforces cultural norms instead of a creating moments to resist the "relation of power in reproduction and sexuality wherein a failure to conceive constitutes a deviation from social norms" (Allison 17). Ironically, although Advocacy Day appears to be resisting the stigmatization of infertility, the strategies, arguments, and narratives RESOLVE petitions attendees to adopt on that day reinforce social norms privileging fertility. Unfortunately, even though RESOLVE attempts to advocate on behalf of infertile women and men so as to "reduce the stigma around infertility and promises to protect legal access to all family building options" ("Infertility Resources"), their activist rhetoric centres on medical discourses of infertility and, at times, reinforces deficit notions of the female body.

QUEERING THE RHETORIC OF INFERTILITY

In pointing to medical discourse as a system to describe, articulate, and study infertility, I draw upon Judith Butler's reflective observation that the "failure to approximate the norm, however, is not the same as the subversion of the norm...there is no promise that subversion will follow from the reiteration of constitutive norm" (23). Given this statement, I ponder what strategies can be deployed to resist and challenge the normalizing heteronormative rhetoric of infertility? Attempting to answer such a question is a large task and needs continued reflection and revision. But to begin the task of resisting the medical discourses of infertility that reinforce deficit attitudes of the infertile female body and to begin creating more critical infertility activist campaigns, I draw upon the queer theory and the discipline of queer studies as it serves as "one method for imaging, not some fantasy of an elsewhere, but existing alternatives to hegemonic systems" (Halberstam 89).

My use of queer theory to destabilize the hegemonic rhetoric of infertility is supported through two aspects of queer scholarship. First, queer studies emerged out of its own activist pursuits by challenging (and continuing to challenge) the normative discourses eroding the possibilities and instabilities of queer. For example,

Michael Warner's *The Trouble with Normal* argues against gay and lesbian activist arguments for marriage equality within the United States. For Warner, the debate over gay marriage in the United States is a debate that fails to address the heart of the issue—the stigmatization of non-normative sex. Warner believes that these activists' attempt to achieve marriage equality does not serve any real advocacy or liberation. His argument influences much of the opposition I express regarding RESOLVE's Advocacy Day. Although on the surface activist discourse may appear to represent the needs of marginalized communities and serve to "break the silence" on such issues, deeper rhetorical examination of the discursive arguments must be performed to fully understand the relationship between the discourse and cultural ideologies.

Second, queer studies does much to resist the regulation of non-normative bodies and non-normative sexualities. Robert McRuer's examination of compulsory able-bodiedness and queer existence serves as an example of the intersectional relationship between queer, non-normative bodies, sexuality, and cultural regulation. Specifically, his work examines the disciplinary structure of normative or able-bodied writing "compulsory able-bodiedness functions by covering over, with the appearance of choice, a system in which there actually is no choice" (491). McRuer elaborates further:

Compulsory heterosexuality functions as a disciplinary formation seemingly emanating from everywhere and nowhere, so too are the origins of able-bodied/disabled identity obscured, allowing for what Susan Wendell calls "the disciplines of normality" to cohere in a system of compulsory able-bodiedness that similarly emanates from everywhere and nowhere. (McRuer 491)

McRuer's point emphasized the importance to critically attend to how bodies are constructed in discourses of "normalcy" and heterosexuality. His statement informs my argument that contemporary scholarship on heteronormative infertility has much to gain and learn from queer theory. Specifically, the experience of infertility actually queers individual understandings of the reproductive-challenged body as no longer a normative body. Additionally, rhetorical discourses of infertility reinforce dominant cultural ideals of heterosexuality. For example, biodmedical discourses frequently employ language promising a sense of hope for the heterosexual infertile couple. In fact, reproductive technologies, such as IVF, serve as a biotechnical solution to reconcile the infertile heterosexual couple to more mainstream cultural norms by allowing them to not only reproduce a biological child of their own but carry that child as well. As such, current rhetorics of infertility fail to make space for more queered and less heterosexual orientations to infertility, profamily legislation, and cultural assumptions of a normative reproductive body.

In *No Future: Queer Theory and the Death Drive*, for example, Lee Edelman adopts a strategically negative stance on what he defines as "reproductive futurism." He asserts the political figure of the child represents the future in which the queer is positioned as the future-negating drive. Specifically, his work highlights the heteronormativity circulating throughout political discourse and legislation that favour the child: "*queerness* names the side of those *not* 'fighting for the children,' the side outside the consensus by which all politics confirms the absolute value of reproductive futurism" (Edelman 3, emphasis in original). Given this, Edelman advocates a queering of such discourse would, instead, embrace this negative subjectivity instead of accommodating a position hailing support for the child. Concerned with the abject negativity of Edelman's position, J. Halberstam writes the following:

> Children, as Edelman would remind us, have been deployed as part of a hetero-logic of futurity or as a link to positive political imaginings of alternatives. But there are alternative productions of the child that recognizes in the image of the nonadult body a propensity to incompetence, a clumsy inability to make sense, a desire for independence for the tyranny of the adult, and a total indifferent to adult conceptions of success and failure. Edelman's negative critique strands queerness between two equally unbearable options (futurity and positivity in opposition to nihilism and negation). Can we produce

generative models of failure that do not posit two equally
bleak alternatives? (120)

For Halberstam, Edelman's position is bleak, too bleak to be fully
embraced. Instead, Halberstam expands on Edelman's position offering a more humanistic approach to failure: "To live is to fail, to
bungle, to disappoint, and ultimately to die; rather than searching
for ways around death and disappointment, the queer art of failure
involves the acceptance of the finite, the embrace of the absurd,
the silly, and the hopelessly goofy" (186-87). So while Edelman's
work exposes the theoretical and discursive gaps within political
and heterosexual discourse, implicitly connecting itself to themes of
infertility previously discussed in this chapter, Halberstam's theory
of failure acts as a more accessible and possible phenomenological
model for a queered intervention to heteronormative infertility:
"While failure certainly comes accompanied by a host of negative
affects, such as disappointment, disillusionment, and despair, it also
provides the opportunity to use these negative affects to poke holes
in the toxic positivity of contemporary life" (Halberstam 3). We
can learn from queer studies how heterosexual infertility is very
much a failure to conform to cultural norms. As a result, feelings
of shame become internalized—noted in the epigraphs included in
the beginning of this chapter—and lead to a sense of stigma and
silence around the topic of infertility.

Yet a queered phenomenological approach to heterosexual infertility may begin to offer a different model in which one may embrace
the reality of such reproductive failure. Queering phenomenology
and attempting to move queer theory toward phenomenology
have great potential, as Sara Ahmed explains: "Phenomenology
can offer a resource for queer studies insofar as it emphasizes the
importance of lived experience, the intentionality of consciousness,
the significance of nearness or what is ready-to-hand, and the role
of repeated and habitual actions in shaping bodies and world" (2).
What results from a queered phenomenology is an account of
"how bodies are gendered, sexualized, and raced by how they
extend into space, as an extension that differentiates between 'left'
and 'right,' 'front' and 'behind,' 'up' and 'down,' as well as 'near'
and 'far'" (Ahmed 5). Although the experience of heteronormative

infertility may not be able to escape the "always, already" disciplinary and discursive rhetoric perpetuating feelings of shame and stigma, the adaptation and continued interdisciplinary scholarship on the intersections between queer theory, infertility, and cultural norms may begin to reorient understandings of infertility. Specifically, the work of queer phenomenology applied to infertility allows for new narratives and new discourses accounting for the embodied realities of heteronormative infertility. Furthermore, as a phenomenology that queers how we are oriented toward particular norms, it serves as a productive exercise to ponder why individuals are oriented toward certain culture desires and affections.

This is a needed framework to be embraced by the infertility community as they grieve their inability to conceive, as well as other infertility stakeholders that counsel and provide support. Queering the rhetoric, the phenomenology, and the narrative of infertility must be adopted beyond an individualistic point-of-view and include more public infertility activist organizations. Infertility advocacy organizations should take steps to reflect on the embedded rhetoric within their campaigns and how language can often reinforce further stigmatization and marginalization.

My hope in writing this piece, as someone who is infertile, is for queer theory to be seen as an ally to evolve the rhetoric of infertility. In this piece, I have tried to illustrate how the experience of infertility continues to be constructed by and through medical discourse. Alternative options—such as living childfree or choosing not to undergo treatment—are not well understood nor are they advocated for. Making visible these alternative narratives can assist in expanding understandings of infertility and shift the rhetoric of infertility, as one that places the female body as an abnormal body, to one that views infertility as a moment to question, confront, and ponder identity. Furthermore, such a shift may allow infertile persons to ponder how and why stigma, shame, and silence surround infertility. Taking time to reflect on what it means to be infertile, rather than try to treat and "fix" infertility, makes space for more critical attention to how medical discourses construct a narrative that to be infertile requires medical treatment, a correction of the abnormal body to a more normal, hetero body. Awareness campaigns that position infertility as a rhetorical sociocultural construct can further shift the scenes and priorities of infertility activism. Rather than perpetuate the medicalization of infertility, perhaps a more effective approach to supporting those living with infertility takes on the system itself: questioning the rhetorical construction of infertility and drawing upon queered discourses to better support the phenomenological moment, or the grappling to understand their body as infertile.

ENDNOTES

[1]My knowledge of RESOLVE's Advocacy Day comes from my own participation in the event. As a cisgendered, heteronormative woman diagnosed with unexplained infertility and a local support volunteer for RESOLVE, I was intrigued by the event and partic-ipated in Advocacy Day in May 2014. Please note that the bills I discuss in this chapter are relevant for a particular year. Historically, what is advocated for during Advocacy Day changes depending upon the current political climate. The example provided here is representative of the 2014 Advocacy Day.

[2]These three bills were selected for the 2014 Advocacy Day.

WORK CITED

Ahmed, Sara. *Queer Phenomenology: Orientations, Objects, Others*. Duke University Press, 2006.

Allison, Jill. "Conceiving Silence: Infertility As Discursive Contra-diction in Ireland." *Medical Anthropology Quarterly*, vol. 25, no. 1, 2011, pp. 1-21.

Althusser, Louis. "Ideology and Ideological State Apparatuses (Notes towards an Investigation)." *Lenin and Philosophy and Other Essays*, (trans. Ben Brewster; New York: Monthly Review Press, 2001 [1971]), pp. 127-86.

Barhite, Brandi. "Groups Help Women Cope with 'Infertility' In-fertility." *Toledo Free Press*, 21 Dec. 2014, issuu.com/toledofree-press/docs/tfp_122114. Accessed 17 Sept. 2017.

Butler, Judith. "Critically Queer." *The Routledge Queer: Studies Reader*, edited by Donald E. Hall et al., Routledge, 2013, pp. 18-31.

Christensen, Jen. "Record Number of Women Using IVF to Get Pregnant—CNN.com." *CNN*, 18 Feb. 2014, http://www.cnn.com/2014/02/17/health/record-ivf-use/. Accessed 13 Sept. 2017.

Edelman, Lee. *No Future: Queer Theory and the Death Drive.* Duke University Press, 2004.

"Fast Facts about Infertility." *RESOLVE: The National Infertility Association*, 6 Apr. 2014, www.resolve.org/about/fast-facts-about-fertility.html. Accessed 13 Sept. 2017.

Foucault, Michel. *The History of Sexuality, Volume I: An Introduction.* Random House, 1990.

Galhardo, A, et al. "The Impact of Shame and Self-Judgment on Psychopathology in Infertile Patients." *Human Reproduction*, vol. 26, no. 9, 2011, pp. 2408-14.

Greil, Arthur, et al. "The Experience of Infertility: a Review of Recent Literature." *Sociology of Health & Illness*, vol. 32, no. 1, 2010, pp. 140-62.

Greil, Arthur. "Infertile Bodies: Medicalization, Metaphor, and Agency." *Infertility Around the Globe: New Thinking on Childlessness, Gender, and Reproductive Technologies*, edited by Marcia C. Inhorn and Frank Van Balen, University of California Press, 2002, pp. 101-18.

Gurunath, S, et al. "Defining Infertility—a Systematic Review of Prevalence Studies." *Human Reproduction Update*, vol. 17, no. 5, 2011, pp. 575-88.

Halberstam, J. *The Queer Art of Failure.* Duke University Press, 2011.

"Infertility Resources." *RESOLVE: The National Infertility Association*, 2017, www.ihr.com/infertility/resources/resolve.html. Accessed 13 Sept. 2017.

Mamo, Laura. *Queering Reproduction: Achieving Pregnancy in the Age of Technoscience.* Duke University Press, 2007.

McRuer, Robert. "Compulsory Able-Bodiedness and Queer/Disabled Existence." *The Routledge Queer: Studies Reader*, edited by Donald E. Hall et al., Routledge, 2013, pp. 488-97.

Pyle, Nate. "The Disgrace of Infertility." *The Huffington Post*, 27 Jan. 2014, www.huffingtonpost.com/nate-pyle/the-disgrace-of-infertility_b_4595151.html. Accessed 13 Sept. 2017.

Sandelowski, Margarete. *With Child in Mind: Studies of the*

Personal Encounter with Infertility. University of Pennsylvania Press, 1993.

Tjørnhøj-Thomsen, Tine. "Close Encounters With Infertility and Procreative Technology." *Managing Uncertainty: Ethnographic Studies of Illness, Risk and the Struggle for* Control, edited by Richard Jenkins, Hanne Jessen and Vibeke Steffen. Museum Tusculanum Press, 2005, pp. 71-91.

Telling Your Story. RESOLVE, 2014.

Warner, Michael. *The Trouble with Normal: Sex, Politics, and the Ethics of Queer Life.* Free Press, 1999.

Whiteford, L.M., and L Gonzalez. "Stigma: the Hidden Burden of Infertility." *Social Science & Medicine*, vol. 40, no. 1, 1995, pp. 27-36.

15.
A Feminist Perspective on Selective Termination

BRITTANY IRVINE

IN REVIEWING the literature on pregnancy loss, I was moved by content, described below, written in Linda Layne's *Motherhood Lost* about a woman's change in identity following a miscarriage ritual. A group of women had gathered to undergo a social rite, which enabled the woman who had experienced the miscarriage to return to work recognized by her social network as no longer pregnant but without a baby. The social rite helped the woman exit from normally sequential identities between pregnancy and motherhood. Although miscarriage is certainly a type of pregnancy loss, it is also a common experience with both formal and informal supports available for women and their partners. On the contrary, loss from selective termination is a rare experience, almost unheard of beyond the maternal fetal medicine community and therefore not socially recognized or understood.

Selective termination complicates the discourse when it comes to pregnancy loss: the subject is no longer pregnant with twins yet will hopefully become a mother of a healthy singleton. She is pregnant with one live fetus and one still fetus and she is facing the simultaneous twin delivery of a stillborn and live born baby. Alternatively, she has had to face a choice to sacrifice her abnormally developing fetus to secure the health of her normally developing one. This is paradoxical—one fetus of a twin pair can survive only if an intervention to terminate the co-fetus occurs. This chapter combines some of the scientific obstetrical literature with the social scientific scholarship on pregnancy loss to contend that a feminist understanding of selective termination is constituted by emphasizing informed choice and shared decision making, and by framing the procedure as an ethically and emotionally complex experience. Approaching this issue from a feminist perspective not only necessitates accounting for the crucial role of scientific information as an enabler of informed choice but also understanding the limitations of communicating about objective perinatal outcomes such as morbidity and mortality. Furthermore, selective termination is one type of termination of pregnancy and hence must be placed in legal and ethical contexts that allow for it. There is also need to better structure clinical care to acknowledge the loss aspects of the procedure during planning and intervention, and during subsequent healthcare encounters, including delivery.

Selective termination is a procedure used to manage high-risk multiples pregnancies, usually twins rather than higher-order multiples such as triplets. The procedure is often confused with fetal reduction. Fetal reduction is the interruption of the development of one or more usually normally developing fetuses in a multiples pregnancy. The intervention is completed in an effort to reduce the number of fetuses in order to reduce maternal, fetal, and infant morbidity and mortality. Literature has demonstrated that higher-order multiples pregnancies, such as triplets and quadruplets, entail greater risk of maternal, fetal, and infant morbidity than twins or singletons, including adverse outcomes from preterm birth (Wen et al.). Thus the process of fetal reduction seeks to reduce morbidity by interrupting the development of one or more fetuses to reduce the pregnancy from high-order multiples to a twin or singleton pregnancy. Fetal reduction usually occurs in the first trimester of pregnancy, and the fetal bodies are reabsorbed into the maternal body and are not delivered (Legendre).

Selective termination is also the interruption of the development of a fetus in a multiples pregnancy, but unlike in fetal reduction, the fetus to be terminated is abnormally developing. It is indicated when one fetus is affected by a serious, incurable pathology and, moreover, when the pathology of the affected fetus could prejudicially affect the healthy development of the co-fetus. Examples of when the procedure has been used include in discordant pregnancies in which one fetus has a congenital anomaly either compatible or incompatible with life or in pregnancies in which the fetuses are

affected by twin-to-twin transfusion syndrome—a complex pathology characterized by disturbances in the blood flow through
a shared placenta (Spadola and Simpson). The terminated fetus
is delivered alongside its co-twin during childbirth, which also
makes the procedure fundamentally different from fetal reduction.

Management strategies for complex twin pregnancies are always
dependent on whether the fetuses at risk are monoamniotic or
diamniotic (i.e., are sharing an amniotic sac or not) and mono-
or di-chorionic (i.e., are sharing a placenta or not). Amniotic sac
and/or placenta sharing depends on the way in which the early
products of conception split, whether in the morula, blastocyst,
or implanted blastocyst stage of development. Fetuses sharing a
placenta can share vascular communication networks. Hence,
the most pressing management concern for these fetuses is that
a spontaneous intrauterine fetal demise of one fetus may trigger
intrauterine fetal demise in the other. Monochorionic monoamniotic
fetuses (i.e., fetuses that share a placenta and an amniotic sac) face
the added risk that they could entangle themselves in their cords,
causing strangulation of one or both of them.

Much of the scientific obstetrical literature on selective termination is in the form of case reports, case series, or meta-analyses.
The body of literature seeks to give a clear estimate of the likelihood of morbidity and mortality of the healthy fetus following
selective termination of the co-fetus. For instance, a study based at
King's College Hospital in London examined the management and
outcomes of eighteen twin pregnancies discordant for anencephaly occurring at their centre, and combined these data with data
from other centres reporting on the same condition. The authors
found that in the dichorionic pregnancies managed with selective
termination, there was one miscarriage of the entire pregnancy,
but 88.9 percent of the pregnancies resulted in live births at a
median gestational age of thirty-seven weeks. In the monochorionic
pregnancies investigated by the researchers, selective termination
resulted in a co-twin survival rate of 77.2 percent and an early
preterm delivery rate of 31.0 percent (Vandecruys et al.). In another study based on eighty cases of selective termination taking
place between 2004 and 2010 at Mount Sinai Medical Center in
New York, the gestational age of the pregnancy at the time of the

selective termination procedure was the only risk factor associated with pregnancy loss and also the only risk factor associated with premature delivery (Bigelow et al.). Other risk factors examined by the study did not reach statistical significance. The authors conclude that selective termination performed earlier in pregnancy is associated with decreased fetal loss of the co-twin and prematurity. This evidence suggests that the decision to proceed with the procedure is time sensitive.

Although these statistics are crucial to informed decision making, they also create a frame implying decisions to selectively terminate should be made based on particular perinatal outcomes, most importantly live birth of the healthy fetus. This becomes the primary outcome lens through which parents are encouraged to assess whether or not to allow both fetuses to continue intrauterine development. There may be other metrics more important to parents though. Understanding the way in which medical literature communicates about this rare procedure is a first step toward a feminist reshaping of the procedure as a pregnancy loss issue. Speaking about statistical significance and statistical associations are important in that they provide information to allow for informed choice, but they miss important aspects of the issue and miscommunicate the complex emotional nature of the choice to proceed with selective termination or not. Although it is important to know that a live birth of the healthy co-fetus is associated with the timing of the procedure and statistically more likely when the procedure happens earlier in gestation, the discourse may be better managed by communicating that the issue is time sensitive and acknowledging that the decision is paradoxical and involves both great loss and the potential for great future joy. Further qualitative research assessing how parents felt about undergoing selective termination could facilitate a more robust understanding about what outcome variables are most important to those for whom the procedure is personal.

Downstream from the selective termination procedure, the stillborn will be delivered alongside a hopefully alive, full-term, healthy baby. The stillborn is often referred to in the medical literature as a papyrus stillborn. How will its parents want to refer to it? Grief for the loss and joy or gratefulness for the live born may exist in parallel at the time of the procedure, at delivery, and in the future. There may be simultaneous grief from having to have made such a choice and joy from the ability to medically manage and intervene to reduce suffering. Notably the terminated fetus may only be partially formed or developmentally anomalous, which may also complicate parental feelings.

Understanding selective termination from a feminist perspective means understanding difficult choices need to be made when selective termination is indicated, and these choices include loss, but they are first and foremost choices for the pregnant woman to make for herself. Informed choice means having the scientific information available to counsel women about the choices available to them and the possible consequences of intervening or not. That is why the scientific literature is so essential to an argument about feminist epistemologies of selective termination. Although the scientific literature has limitations with respect to how it accounts for simultaneous emotions, without the scientific information about risks and outcomes, informed choice would not be possible. Whether a choice, informed or otherwise, is an option at all depends on termination procedures being legal and accessible.

A feminist perspective on this pregnancy loss issue necessitates discussion of a woman's right to choose termination of her pregnancy. One study on selective termination discussed cases of twin pregnancies wherein each fetal pair was discordant for lethal open cranial defects (Sepulvada et al.). In one case, though the anomalous fetus was not going to survive outside the womb and was a risk to the continued development of the co-twin, the mother had to be referred to a fetal surgery centre in the United States. The selective termination procedure was illegal in Chile. Termination was not available in Chile even though the procedure may have ensured the viability of the co-twin and its continued normal development. In contrast, a second case featured in the study took place in Argentina. Although Argentinian law also prohibits elective termination of pregnancy, the particular case was taken to local ethics and legal committees for approvals; it was advocated for based on the fact that the selective termination aimed to improve the perinatal outcomes of the normally developing fetus. Both of these cases resulted in live births of the normally developing co-fetuses at near and full term, respectively. The third case summarized in the study (also based in Chile) had a different outcome. In that case, although the parents desired selective termination, an independent ethics committee did not approve the procedure. Finances limited the parents from seeking treatment internationally. At twenty-five weeks' gestation, intrauterine fetal demise of the normally developing twin was observed, with the anencephalic fetus maintaining a heartbeat. It died soon after it was delivered.

This case series reports how selective termination can dramatically change a prognosis but also demonstrates how antichoice legislation can threaten fetal viability. Furthermore, this case series is a welcome reminder of the myriad medical contexts in which termination is an option. The right to choice must be legally enshrined, in part, to ensure the choice to selectively terminate one fetus for the sake of another. Before discussions on informed choice and shared decision making are truly relevant, the right to choice must be enshrined.

Thus far I have argued that a feminist perspective on selective termination has two pillars: acknowledgment that the scientific literature has limitations but is necessary to facilitate informed choice; and that choice to electively terminate pregnancy remains the background context upon which selective termination is possible. The third pillar of this feminist perspective is facilitating action to enhance the choice process, structure the continuum of care as parents wish, and acknowledge the pregnancy loss aspects of the procedure and its effects. Shared decision making may help in this regard.

Shared decision making is a process by which patients and healthcare providers make a treatment decision taking into account the patient's perspective, preferences, and values and accounts for the best available evidence of treatment options. Numerous studies I reviewed wrote that parents were counselled before they made a decision to move forward with selective termination. This counselling could be enhanced if it was revisited at particular points along the continuum of care and if the numerous loss aspects involved in the decision making were taken into account during these counselling sessions. For instance, counselling could begin when clinicians find the affected pregnancy. It could continue before and after the selective termination procedure, and it could continue before the delivery and into the postpartum period. It could acknowledge the loss of normalcy parents are facing. The popular discourse of what childbirth should be like is certainly inapplicable for women who have undergone selective termination. Instead the discourse could acknowledge the simultaneous grief and joy parents may be facing by addressing these emotions directly. Using phrases and words that show parents they are the ones who are able to decide how they wish their terminated fetus to be referred to in subsequent healthcare encounters and at the delivery could help. Further research into how best to engage clinicians and patients in shared decision making around selective termination is needed.

Best practices during delivery would include showing empathy and kindness to the woman and her family, and using the terms they have chosen to acknowledge their babies and their complex emotional and ethical situation. Prior to delivery asking the family what protocols they would like followed during the birth, including whether or not they wish to see their stillborn, could help contour these life changing moments to align with the woman and her family's values and preferences. In their article on good practices when dealing with perinatal death, Alix Henley and Judith Schoot write that although "it may be clinically correct to talk about the 'products of conception' ... most parents talk about their 'baby' from the beginning of the pregnancy" (326). This idea is echoed in other literature as well. Linda Layne, in her article "Breaking the Silence," quotes a woman saying that "for many women ... the child begins when the decision is made to bear it" (8). Layne also acknowledges the inherent tensions involved in acknowledging the loss of a fetus while not prescribing the fetus personhood. For a feminist perspective of pregnancy loss, one must be able to do both: acknowledge the loss and ascribe women the right to choose. For a feminist perspective on selective termination to be actualized, one must be able to choose the procedure based on scientific information, acknowledge the limitations of that information, and practice shared decision making to better contour the experience to the values and preferences of the family who will face the consequences of their choices for a lifetime.

WORKS CITED

Bigelow, Catherine, et al. "Timing of and Outcomes After Selective Termination of Anomalous Fetuses in Dichorionic Twin Pregnancies." *Prenatal Diagnosis,* vol. 34, no. 13, 2014, pp. 1320-25.

Henley, Alix, and Judith Schott. "The Death of a Baby Before, During or Shortly after Birth: Good Practice from the Parents' Perspective." *Seminars in Fetal and Neonatal Medicine*, vol. 13, no. 5, 2008, pp. 325-28.

Layne, Linda. "Breaking the Silence: An Agenda for a Feminist Discourse of Pregnancy Loss." *Feminist Studies*, vol. 23, no. 2, 1997, pp. 289-315.

Layne, Linda. *Motherhood Lost: A Feminist Account of Pregnancy Loss in America.* Routledge, 2003.

Legendre, Claire-Marie, et al. "Differences between Selective Termination of Pregnancy and Fetal Reduction in Multiple Pregnancy: A Narrative Review." *Reproductive BioMedicine Online*, vol. 26, no. 6, pp. 542-54.

Sepulveda, Waldo, et al. "Monoamniotic Twin Pregnancy Discordant for Lethal Open Cranial Defect: Management Dilemmas." *Prenatal Diagnosis*, vol. 3, no. 6, 2013, pp. 578-82.

Spadola, Alexandra, and Lynn Simpson. "Selective Termination Procedures in Monochorionic Pregnancies." *Seminars in Perinatology*, vol. 29, no. 5, 2005, pp. 330-37.

Vandecruys et al. "Dilemmas in the Management of Twins Discordant For Anencephaly Diagnosed at 11+0 to 13+6 weeks of Gestation." *Ultrasound in Obstetrics and Gynecology*, vol. 28, no. 2, 2006, pp. 653-58.

Wen, Shi Wu, et al. "Maternal Morbidity and Obstetric Complications in Triplet Pregnancies and Quadruplet and High-Order Multiple Pregnancies." *American Journal of Obstetrics and Gynecology*, vol. 191, no. 1, 2004, pp. 254-58.

V. MEMORIALIZING LOSS

16.
Enacting Acknowledgement, Meaning, and Acceptance

Personal Ceremony and Ritual as Helpful Ways to Engage with Feelings of Loss after Abortion

MIRIAM ROSE BROOKER

THIS CHAPTER EXPLORES accounts of the ceremonial and ritual expressions of three Australian women who grieved the pregnancies they ended through elective abortion,[1] and is interwoven with broader research findings about the usefulness of ritual for engaging with loss. These three women took part in my larger PhD research study about how women come to terms with the complexity and challenges often accompanying ending a pregnancy. The phenomenologically grounded research methodology employed in the study proceeded in two phases and was designed to access the ways in which women generate meaning about their abortion experiences through stories and their bodily-felt senses. The first phase, including twenty-three Australian women, invited each participant to retell her abortion experiences and how she interpreted them via an open-ended, semistructured personal interview, an online survey, or a journal. The second phase included eight women from phase one, who returned to participate in an innovative focusing and art process designed to access each woman's subjective bodily-felt sense of her abortion experiences (Brooker). Not all women perceive having an abortion as a loss, but about half of my participants did so, and they tended to grieve the aborted being and the opportunity to mother.

I asked participants if they had conducted a ceremony or a ritual in relation to their abortion as part of a larger research question about what the time after the abortion was like for them, or how they coped. Four interview participants out of seventeen and two out of six anonymous online survey or journal partici-

209

pants reported engaging in a ceremony or ritual. Three of these participants provided brief details: one planted memorial trees and said some prayers for her two aborted children[2]; another described herself as pagan and held a "release and self-forgiveness" ritual, which included a meditation to go back and interact with her preabortion self (to let her know that it was okay); and the third conducted a simple ritual on the beach to acknowledge that she had an abortion. However, this chapter focuses on three interview participants who provided more detail about what their ceremony or ritual had involved, what it meant to them, and how it had helped them. I argue that the rich symbols and gestures these three women engaged with characterize the ways in which they actively made sense of and acknowledged their experiences of loss after abortion.

My participants discerned for themselves if they held a ceremony or ritual after abortion, and their examples shape the way that ceremony and ritual are presented within this chapter. Their ceremonial and ritual expressions were unique to them, and they occurred as part of a one-off and out-of-the-ordinary event. They used symbols and gestures representing their active and embodied attempts to come to terms with their abortion or to acknowledge the lost potential being. My participants' ceremonial and ritual expressions all emphasized the personal meaning of their abortion or loss rather than any social processes of being witnessed or of trying to express meaning or significance to anyone who happened to be present.

The ways these three participants developed or expressed ceremony and ritual incorporated personally meaningful, symbolic, and intentional words or actions. The rituals were performed after abortion, and they acknowledged the potential being that was lost or helped to reconcile their challenging feelings and beliefs about having had an abortion. Thus, their expressions of ceremony and ritual align with the ways that ritual was developed and expressed in feminist spiritual support groups during the 1990s. Diann Neu has identified that feminist group rituals offered "women an important buffer to change, [and] a way of consciously recognizing and supporting a life event rather than denying it or rejecting it" (191). Neu acknowledges the lack of rituals for the transitions that occur within women's life cycles, including abortion, and sees it as an important role for feminists to create these "new ceremonies of transition" (Neu 192). Although my participants have largely developed their own ceremonial and ritual expressions, they share qualities with the ways that women have been observed to engage in ritual making more generally. After researching women's contemporary ritual development and performance, Jan Berry defines ritual-making as a "strategic practice that women choose to negotiate the changes and transitions in their lives. It makes creative use of symbol and space to interpret and construct not only experience, but theo/alogy[3] and spirituality" (Berry 129). Despite definitional differences in the way that the term "ritual" is used, within this chapter, I have referred to the broader academic literature on ritual in which its personal benefits, particularly in the context of a loss, are emphasized.

HOW CEREMONY AND RITUAL CAN ENGAGE WITH LOSS

Erin's[4] decision to have an abortion was not straight forward, since her initial response to the pregnancy was happiness and a strong sense of wanting to keep the baby.[5] She explained her conflict as follows: "when it was just me I felt a really strong connection with being pregnant. I kept on going, 'This can work, this can work,' but with me and Mike,[6] every time he was there or every time I thought about him, it was just like it wasn't working, it wasn't working." Erin said that she did not think abortion was the right thing, and she initially perceived it as an "act against life or an act against a process." She said that she saw herself as someone who had always "gone with the flow" and she acknowledged her abortion decision to be the first time she had actively halted a process by saying "no."

The Australian crow is native to Northern and Western Australia, and it became a strong symbol for Erin, as she deliberated on and came to terms with her abortion decision. During the interview, Erin told me about a visit she made to one of her special places in nature—the same lake where she was sitting when she first realized that she was pregnant. She was waiting there to tell Mike she was pregnant when she saw a crow:

211

I was sitting by the lake and this crow came and sat in the branch, maybe just a metre and a half above my head, and it was carrying an egg in its beak and it was just staring at me like nothing I've really experienced before. Just staring at me, and then it flew off over the lake with the egg and I always think back to what that might mean ... one part of me thinks that it was never supposed to be and it was like the crow going, "It's not for you now," [and] taking it off in a way.

Erin felt the crow symbolized a timely end to her pregnancy, but she also told me that she felt the crow could be warning her that she should be careful with this one chance because it might be taken away. Erin resolved this conflict after her abortion had taken place when she witnessed an Aboriginal legend relating to the local area being reenacted. In the story, a man's son died, and his spirit was carried to the other side by a crow. Erin remembered having a strong emotional response to hearing the legend: "it just made me cry and cry and cry because I just, I just kind of felt like the crows were there to take, to help and to take the spirit and that just helped me realize that there was deeper things going on, or that there was support in other realms." Although Erin is not Indigenous, she has developed strong affiliations with local Aboriginal people and has engaged deeply with their culture and traditions. Thus, an Indigenous and land-connected retelling helped her to affirm the supportiveness of the crow with the egg. She also accessed a sense of the existential help and reassurance that was there for the spirit of the fetus and, ultimately, for herself.

Erin let her body guide her to bring her pregnancy and abortion experience full circle. She requested to receive the ashes of the aborted fetus after her procedure. These were given to her in a little box with a butterfly on top of it. As she drove past her special lake on the way home, she felt moved to stop the car and get out:

The sun was setting in this particular way, and there was all this kind of light and kind of rainbow-ish kind of light and I just, it was like my body just did it. I just got out of the car and kind of waded into the lake a bit and put the ashes in there and it kind of felt nice because it was where I first realized [that I was pregnant] and [it was]where the crow was, and I've always had a special love of that lake and so I felt really good.

Erin's ritual actions took place in a natural environment that she loved, at sunset, surrounded by a rainbow-like light. Her description of her ritual actions evokes a sense of beauty and peace around the ending of her pregnancy.

The experiences of my participants indicate that women can derive a range of benefits from engaging with personal ritual. One of these benefits is described by James Clarke as "balanced emotional expression." According to Clarke, ritual works to both contain and sustain emotion within its rhythmic dance of both acknowledging intense emotion and letting it go. An important component of being able to release emotion and reframe a loss is a combination of both being involved in the ritual and being able to hold the awareness of an observer (Kirmayer). This means striking a balance between feeling emotionally overwhelmed and separating from the loss experience. Conducting ritual can also evoke a sense of safety or sacredness, which helps this emotional balance to be maintained (Kirmayer). Ritual may also help by reducing difficult emotional experiences while increasing positive ones, including relief (Norton and Gino).

At one point during her interview Erin stated, "I remember quite a few times like I'd made the wrong choice and not knowing how I'd ever, ever, ever reconcile myself. I felt like I never ever would." Her comment is resonant with grief and self-doubt, which in Erin's case centred on the loss of the opportunity to mother a baby at that time. However, engaging with ritual and symbolism helped her to transform the way she thought about and related to the aborted fetus. She came to acknowledge it as a being that is part of nature and that is supported spiritually, beyond the physical realm. From this existential perspective, Erin could access more peace in relation to her abortion decision.

New ways of being with loss can be enacted through the body as it moves mindfully and symbolically through ritual. When she instinctively stopped by the lake, Erin's body moved to find resolution through ritual action. She deliberately spread the ashes of the fetus out on the water of the lake, physically and symbolically letting it go back into nature. Ritual helps to connect embodied knowing with intentional action (Clarke). Performing ritual with the body can help a person feel as though they are doing something to help themselves in a situation that has left them feeling powerless or overwhelmed (Rando). In addition, enacting ritual can help a person to reconnect with a fuller sense of their loss rather than being caught up in their mind's limiting analysis of it (Rando). The body can guide this in a way that is not emotionally overwhelming. Therese Rando observes that ritual "is not merely a reflection of meaning but can also be a way of shaping meanings" (Rando 121). Erin's ritual actions made it possible for the lost fetus to be released and to become part of one of her special places in nature. Symbolism and ritual helped her to engage with strong emotions and existential themes, as her mind and her body worked together to find resolution.

WHEN ABORTION IS FELT AS A LOSS

Melissa needed a way to come to terms with her intense feelings of loss, grief, and guilt after a late-term abortion. Her mental health caseworker approached me to see if Melissa could participate in my research because she hoped Melissa might find some closure by telling her abortion story. To facilitate this, Melissa's caseworker provided a special interview space for Melissa and me to share, which was adorned with flowers, incense, and a candle. Thus, the telling of the story became a ritual process. During the interview, Melissa recounted how when another family member had an abortion, her own numbness started to dissipate and she began to feel upset. She then went and looked online at information about the medical procedure, which she said intensified her feelings of guilt and regret in relation to the aborted fetus. She acknowledged, "Yeah, I just feel guilt, regret, and I just want to know that it's in a nice place [Melissa cried]."

Women's emotional responses to abortion are not always straightforward, since they can involve a mixture of both positive and more challenging feelings. Such feelings can be both complex and multilayered. For example, it is common for women to know they made the right decision to have the abortion and to also experience painful feelings. A Swedish research study (Kero et al.) illustrates this well. They found that the majority of their fifty-eight interview participants, one year after having an abortion, experienced the abortion as an expression of responsibility, maturity, and relief. However, half of their participants also experienced difficult feelings alongside these more positive feeling experiences. Of the twenty-nine women who experienced mixed feelings about a past abortion, the most common words they chose to express their painful feelings were grief, injustice, guilt and emptiness (Kero, Högberg and Lalos).

Grieving after abortion can be a disconcerting experience, particularly when a woman's ideological positioning is at odds with her emotional responses (Keys). For example, prochoice women are more likely to experience their abortion as a relief, yet feelings such as loss, grief, and guilt may also emerge over time. This kind of ideological-emotional discordance can be challenging:

> Prochoice women ... subscribe to an entirely different set of beliefs. For them, feeling or expressing anything other than the proscribed [sic] relief can be troubling. But even when there are no gaps, prochoice women may still need to engage in emotion work to maintain the desired emotion, to reduce anxiety or pain, or to deflect negative characterizations and attempts by others to personify the fetus. (Keys 64)

Experiencing abortion as a loss may prompt women to seek ways to acknowledge and express their complex and multilayered responses to abortion.

When women experience abortion as a loss, these feelings can persist for years if they are not acknowledged. For example, a research study conducted in the United States demonstrates that low levels of grief were still present for the eighty-three participants up to twenty-six years later (Williams). In a Norwegian follow-up study, the mental health outcomes of miscarriage were compared with those for abortion. These researchers found that feelings of loss and guilt lessened significantly over the time following a miscarriage, but not an abortion (Broen et al.). The social context surrounding a woman having an abortion may not acknowledge that she has a right to grieve that loss because "every society has norms that frame grieving" (Doka, "Disenfranchised" 225). Those rules dictate which losses are considered legitimate and whether or not others will offer sympathy or support. Women are not expected to grieve after abortion when having the abortion is a choice or when abortion looks like a logical solution to a challenging pregnancy situation. Without a framework for understanding grief and loss after abortion, women are left to decipher their feelings alone. They may carry a sense of personal or moral responsibility obscuring the social and relational context that influenced their situation as well as their personal responses for having an abortion. Although prolife discourses encourage women to see the fetus as a baby and abortion as the loss of a life, they also frame abortion as a moral shortcoming (Mason), and this can leave women carrying residual feelings that are difficult to resolve.

Thinking of the pregnancy as containing a child can contribute to feelings of loss after abortion. Maria Stålhandske and colleagues found that 67 percent of their Swedish survey participants reported thinking about the child lost as a result of an abortion (Stålhandske et al.). They found that thinking about the fetus as a child, having spiritual beliefs, and engaging with existential thoughts and practices were interrelated. Women engaging with more existential considerations of "morality, identity, meaning and mortality" were also more likely to describe the decision to abort as difficult and to experience lower levels of psychological wellbeing (Stålhandske et al. 54).

Alongside thinking about the pregnancy in terms of a child, my research findings suggest that having children before or after an abortion can contribute to feelings of loss. Women's experiences of pregnancy and motherhood can give them a different frame of reference for what an abortion means to them. Melissa reported that having another child after her abortion contributed to her heightened feelings of grief and guilt. After her next baby was born, she realized that she could cope, since she felt spiritually and mentally stronger, and this led her to regret the earlier abortion: "I think also because if I wasn't to go on and have more children after I don't think I'd hold so much guilt. And I think because I went and had children after, and because I'm dealing with their father, you know, that's where the guilt comes, because I could have done it and I know now that I could have done it." In addition to feeling more resourceful, Melissa reported that she appreciated children a lot more: "after that abortion, I look at children differently. All of them, they're just so innocent and beautiful, I'm more clucky, I've definitely been more clucky." Having an abortion and considering that pregnancy in human terms led to Melissa's heightened valuing of her next pregnancy and child. Conversely, for women who have an abortion after having children, the abortion can represent the loss of another opportunity to be a mother or to relate with a "child that could not be" (Nathanson 218).

Women who experience their abortion as a loss may continue to grieve because their feelings are unacknowledged or discounted. Melissa told me that she was disconcerted to find her family and friends simply expected her to move on with her life after her abortion, whereas she felt really shaken up by it. Beverley Raphael notes that women are often expected to feel grateful after obtaining an abortion or to experience relief, since the problem of unwanted pregnancy has been rectified. She also identifies that there is little support or general knowledge available about coping with the to-and-fro feelings women can experience in response to having an induced abortion.

Kenneth Doka's concept of "disengranchised grief" is a helpful way of thinking about the mismatch that can occur between women's experiences of loss after abortion and social expectations. Doka defines disenfranchised grief as follows

> grief that results when a person experiences a signficant loss and the resultant grief is not openly acknowledged, socially validated, or publicly mourned. In short, although the individual is experiencing a grief reaction, there is no social recognition that the person has a right to grieve or a claim for social sympathy or support. (Doka "Disenfranchised Grief in Historical and Cultural Perspective" 224)

The personal significance of having an abortion can also be disenfranchised by medical approaches and practices emphasizing a quick return to normality or those that are overly cold and clinical (Aléx and Hammarström). Lena Aléx and Anne Hammarström emphasize the importance of medical personnel taking account of women's complex experiences throughout the process of having an abortion, including afterward. Women need encouragement and support to experience and come to terms with any feelings that arise for them. According to Doka, ritual is a good way of acknowledging and addressing diverse experiences of loss and, in particular, disenfranchised grief (Doka "The Role of Ritual in the Treatment of Disenfranchised Grief").

During the interview, ritual emerged as a good way for Melissa to come to terms with her intense feelings about her abortion. Following our interview, Melissa's caseworker suggested her ritual might take the form of a "letting go ceremony," and Melissa later sent me a written account of her experience. She had enacted her letting go ceremony at her local beach, which was a special place for her:

> I went to the spot where I was baptised because that's close to my heart. I took flowers. There was one white one that washed up on the shore that resembled peace to me. I took a butterfly and put it in the sand under the water because for me butterflies resemble the free spirit. I prayed to god to tell my baby that I love the little one and that I'm sorry and that I will love it forever. I asked god to show me a sign that my baby heard me, then left and walked up to the swings where my other children were playing with my case worker. My daughter came up to me and showed me a ring that a little girl had just given her ... it was a butterfly ring. That was my sign. When the children were young I always used lavender baby bath. I took some down and tipped it into the ocean. To me this was the looking after and caring for that I never got to do, and lavender helps you to sleep well. Now I accept that my baby is in a world of no pain, just love and light ... one day I will be with my baby ... I am now letting

go of the guilt and sorrow. As god forgives me, I learn to forgive myself and others.

Melissa's ritual was enacted in a natural place she loved and that was already spiritually significant to her. Her ritual actions were steeped in symbolism and meaning, and her gestures of caring and letting go helped her to find some reassurance and comfort. Melissa's personal ritual allowed her to acknowledge and own her experiences of what it meant to have an abortion, despite the contrary beliefs and expectations of her family and friends.

CEREMONY AND RITUAL AS SYMBOLIC ACTION AFTER ABORTION

Some women are drawn to ritual as a meaningful way of acknowledging and engaging with their personal feelings of loss after an abortion. Stålhandske and colleagues found that nearly half of their participants (48 percent) "reported that they had conducted, or had wanted to conduct, a special act to mark the end of the process, or to be reconciled with the event" of abortion (Stålhandske et al. 56). Neu acknowledges that a key aspect of ritual is connective and one way it achieves this is through the "integration of the self with itself" (Neu 191).

My participants engaged symbolically with items and aspects of nature readily available to them and in ways reflecting to themselves deeply resonant layers of meaning and significance. Erin found that the crow, a sunset, and a lake spoke deeply to her inner sense of her abortion experience, whereas Melissa found meaning in flowers, butterflies, and lavender baby bath. They also used gestures to symbolize releasing or letting go of the baby or the difficult emotional aspects of their abortion experiences. The symbols women choose to represent and express their inner understandings about an abortion experience have the power to communicate beyond words. As Victor Turner has noted, symbols communicate multiple meanings simultaneously, since "A single symbol, in fact, represents many things at the same time: it is multivocal, not univocal" (Turner 52).

The Japanese Buddhist ritual for perinatal loss, *Mizuko Kuyō*, uses the symbol of an infant in a way that conveys connection, protection, and blessing. As Elizabeth Harrison depicts it, the purpose of the ritual (translated as "water child" ritual) is to help parents who have miscarried or aborted a pregnancy to (re)establish a relationship with their mizuko (dead or unseen child(ren)) (Harrison and Midori). Within Japan, the ritual of Mizuko Kuyō can include purchasing an infant-like statue of Jizō, the bodhisattva who suffers for others and who protects children; and dressing it in baby clothes, wrapping it in a blanket, adorning it with small toys and flowers, or surrounding it with toys, pinwheels, or food (Harrison and Midori; Klass and Heath). The form of the ceremony varies across temples in Japan but includes the key elements of naming the dead child and giving it form to acknowledge its existence (Harrison and Midori).

Reilly took part in a group Mizuko Kuyō ritual for women who had lost babies through stillbirth and miscarriage, and found herself symbolically acknowledging a previous abortion too. Although she went along with the intention of mourning the stillbirth of one of her children, she also found herself spontaneously naming a fetus she had aborted fifteen years previously:

> And that ceremony then became ... my little abortion ceremony type of thing, and I don't think I actually planned it that way but it rose out of that moment and ... that's the time I named the baby.... it became a real baby type thing, not that it was ever a baby, but it really was, you have your own children by the end so it becomes even more, the loss, that it's a child, that it was yours, it was more acknowledged.

For Reilly, the symbolic action of naming her "unseen" aborted child allowed her to recognize its place in her life and to make its existence more real. Through the Mizuko Kuyō ritual, she could be more present with her sadness and regret about that lost child. The place where Reilly's ritual was held, a local beach cove, has since become one of her special places to visit and remember her lost children. It has become invested with significance and meaning for her.

The Mizuko Kuyō ceremony gave Reilly the opportunity to ackowledge both of her lost babies with equal validity. As part of my research, I spoke with the Buddhist nun, Cate Juno, who facilitated Reilly's ceremony. Juno has offered the Mizuko Kuyō ritual as a way of addressing the isolation, loss, and shame that Australian women can experience around having had an abortion, since from a Buddhist perpective no distinction is made between miscarriage, stillbirth, or abortion. Reilly found this approach very reassuring and affirming, since her feeling of loss in relation to her abortion had been deepening as time passed.

SUMMARY AND CONCLUSION

Each of these women engaged with ritual symbols and gestures in a way that brought her a sense of acknowledgment, completion, acceptance, or forgiveness, as appropriate to her personal need. They all contacted a broader spiritual or existential framework through ritual, which helped them to reframe their abortion experiences in ways that were more compassionate or reasuring for them.

It is interesting that the ritual examples provided in this chapter occurred outdoors and near bodies of water. Water absorbs, cleanses, reflects, sooths, dissolves, and transforms. For these women it facilitated the emotional process of being with and releasing feelings of loss after abortion. Each of my participants derived support and reassurance through her interactions with the watery environment where her ritual took place.

It's also apparent that none of these women started with a planned script or series of actions. Rather, they interacted with the external environment in ways that allowed their insights and meanings about their abortions to develop and unfold in a kindly way. It was by chance that the white flower was the one that came back toward Melissa on a sea wave, which then symbolized peace returning to her. It was only later when Erin witnessed the reinacment of a story involving a crow that she accepted her crow to be benevolent and supportive. Reilly did not intend to name the aborted fetus at her Mizuko Kuyō ritual, but naming and mourning her stillborn baby opened this opportunity. The bodily aspect of all three experiences needs to be acknowledged, since the body continues to live, experience, and process, and its ongoing interactions with the environment and symbolism helped each woman to make sense of an abortion experience they found unsettling and challenging. It is remarkable that these three women could evoke so much peace, significance, and meaning around what was a problematic ending of a pregnancy for each of them. Ceremony, ritual, and symbolism, when enacted in this self-speaking-to-itself way, has the power to transform how women feel about their abortion experiences and themselves.

For some women ritual is a powerful way of acknowleding and coming to terms with conflicted feelings about a past abortion and of recognizing, connecting with, or expressing care for the aborted being. Because of the lack of spaces, opportunities, or culturally sanctioned ways for Western women to engage with abortion as a loss, some turn to personal ceremony and ritual as a way of doing so. Feminist spiritual groups and practitioners have long encouraged women to acknowledge, own, and express their significant lifecycle transitions and experiences through ritual. Some contemporary women are now moved to develop their own private, ceremonial, and ritual expressions, or to draw upon rituals from other cultures after having an abortion. Engaging symbolically and ritually is an active, creative, and embodied way for women to cope with and come to terms with personal experiences of loss after abortion.

ENDNOTES

[1] In this chapter, I use the term "abortion" rather than termination because that is the word the women in this chapter used.

[2] "Children" is the term that this participant used to refer to her aborted fetuses. Throughout this chapter, I have used the terminology of my participants to refer to the potential life terminated with the pregnancy.

[3] A discourse that reflects on the meaning of God (theo) or Goddess (thea).

[4] Not her real name. All participants chose their own pseudonym within the research.

[5] "Baby" is the term that this participant used to refer to the fetus.

[6] Not his real name.

WORKS CITED

Aléx, Lena, and Anne Hammarström. "Women's Experiences in Connection with Induced Abortion–a Feminist Perspective." *Scandinavian Journal of Caring Sciences,* vol. 18, no. 2, 2004, pp. 160-68.

Berry, Jan. *Ritual Making Women: Shaping Rites for Changing Lives.* Equinox Publishing, 2009.

Broen, A.N., et al. "The Course of Mental Health after Miscarriage and Induced Abortion: A Longitudinal, Five-Year Follow-up Study." *BMC Medicine,* vol. 3, no. 1, 2005, pp. 18.

Brooker, Miriam Rose. "Focusing and Artistic Expression as Ways to Explore the Implicit and Non-Verbal Aspects of Women's Abortion Experiences." *Outskirts,* vol. 32, pp. 1-14.

Clarke, James J. Ritual: *A Mythic Means of Personal and Social Transformation.* Pacifica Graduate Institute, 2008.

Doka, Kenneth J. "Disenfranchised Grief in Historical and Cultural Perspective." *Handbook of Bereavement Research and Practice: Advances in Theory and Intervention,* edited by Margaret Stroeve et al., American Psychological Association, 2008, pp. 223-40.

Doka, Kenneth J. "The Role of Ritual in the Treatment of Disenfranchised Grief." *Disenfranchised Grief: New Directions, Challenges, and Strategies for Practice,* edited by Kenneth J. Doka, Research Pub, 2002, pp. 135-47.

Harrison, E G, and I Midori. "Women's Responses to Child Loss in Japan: The Case of" Mizuko Kuyō [with Response]." *Journal of Feminist Studies in Religion,* vol. 11, no. 2, 1995, pp. 67-100.

Juno, Cate Kodo. "Healing a Lost Pregnancy." *Nova: Australia's Holistic Journal,* vol. 6-7, 2014, novaholisticjournal.com/stories/ healing-a-lost-pregnancy. Accessed 17 Sept. 2017.

Kero, Anneli, et al. "Wellbeing and Mental Growth—Long-Term Effects of Legal Abortion." *Social Science & Medicine,* vol. 58, no. 12, 2004, pp. 2559-569.

Keys, Jennifer. "Running the Gauntlet: Women's Use of Emotion Management Techniques in the Abortion Experience." *Symbolic Interaction,* vol. 33, no. 1, 2010, pp. 41-70.

Kirmayer, Laurence J. "The Cultural Diversity of Healing: Meaning, Metaphor and Mechanism." *British Medical Bulletin,* vol.

69, no. 1, 2004, pp. 33-48.

Klass, Dennis, and Amy Olwen Heath. "Grief and Abortion: Mizu-ko Kuyo, the Japanese Ritual Resolution." *OMEGA-Journal of Death and Dying*, vol. 34, no. 1, 1997, pp. 1-14.

Mason, Carol. *Killing for Life: The Apocalyptic Narrative of Pro-Life Politics*. Cornell University Press, 2002.

Nathanson, Sue. *Soul Crisis: One Woman's Journey through Abortion to Renewal*. New American Library, 1989.

Neu, Diann. "Women's Empowerment through Feminist Rituals." *Women & Therapy*, vol. 16, no 2-3, 1995, pp.185-200.

Norton, Michael I, and Francesca Gino. "Rituals Alleviate Grieving for Loved Ones, Lovers, and Lotteries." *Journal of Experimental Psychology*, vol. 143, no. 1, 2014, pp. 266-72.

Rando, Therese A. "Creating Therapeutic Rituals in the Psycho-therapy of the Bereaved." *Psychotherapy: Theory, Research, Practice, Training*, vol. 22, no. 2, 1985, pp. 236-40.

Raphael, Beverley. *The Anatomy of Bereavement*. Hutchinson and Co, 1984.

Stålhandske, Maria Liljas, et al. "Existential Experiences and Needs Related to Induced Abortion in a Group of Swedish Women: A Quantitative Investigation." *Journal of Psychosomatic Obstetrics & Gynecology*, vol. 33, no. 2, 2012, pp. 53-61.

Turner, Victor W. *The Ritual Process: Structure and Anti-Structure*. Aldine Publishing Company, 1969.

Williams, Gail. "Grief after Elective Abortion: Exploring Nursing Interventions for Another Kind of Perinatal Loss." *AWHONN Lifelines*, vol. 4, no. 2, 2000, pp. 37-40.

17.
Queering Reproductive Loss

Exploring Grief and Memorialization

CHRISTA CRAVEN AND ELIZABETH PEEL

L ESBIAN, GAY, BISEXUAL, transgender, and queer (LGBTQ) communities have a long history of memorializing loss—The NAMES Project or AIDS memorial quilt, the Transgender Day of Remembrance, and art and fiction memorializing the Stonewall riots. Yet as Heather Love cautions in *Feeling Backward*, queer losses are frequently hard to identify or mourn since many aspects of historical gay culture are associated with the pain and shame of the closet (2). The subject of reproductive loss—the personal, and sometimes communal, experiences of miscarriage, infant death, and failed adoptions—has often been a silent burden for LGBTQ parents, one frequently intensified by fears of homophobia and heterosexism. Queer losses are also overlooked (or perhaps avoided) in most academic and popular books on LGBTQ reproduction, and queer experiences remain absent from most self-help books on recovering from reproductive loss (Peel and Cain).

J. Halberstam has argued that "failure" to meet conventional standards of success (in this case bringing children into a family, albeit a queer one) can offer creative, cooperative, and surprising ways of challenging heteronormative understandings of love and life (2). Furthermore, Juana María Rodríguez advocates a reconceptualization of a queer sexual politics informed by both utopian longings and everyday failures (7). This chapter takes up the everyday experiences of queer reproductive losses and the memorialization of these experiences through physical memorials, religious and/or spiritual services, and commemorative tattoos.

The personal narratives and photographs included in this chapter are drawn from survey and interview data from LGBTQ parents gathered by two researchers—an American anthropologist and a British psychologist—who met online after their own experiences with pregnancy loss as queer women. Christa and her partner lost a baby in 2009 at eighteen weeks, and Elizabeth and her partner experienced a "silent" miscarriage at twelve weeks in 2008 (Peel and Cain). We found few resources to help us cope with loss in queer families.

We have collected the stories of queer people—primarily lesbian and bisexual women, but also several gay men and trans people—about their experiences of reproductive loss. These stories are drawn from an online survey of sixty non-heterosexual women from the UK, USA, Canada, and Australia (Peel), and interviews with fifty-two LGBTQ people who had experienced loss in the USA, Canada, and a handful of other countries, including Belgium, Italy, Jamaica, New Zealand, and Scotland. Elsewhere, we have argued that for LGBTQ people, challenges in achieving conception and adoption amplify experiences of loss and the severely under-researched experiences of non-gestational parents[1] offer important insights into the range of experience with reproductive loss (Craven and Peel). We reengage that conversation here: first, in the existing literature on reproductive loss in queer communities; second, in the (lack of) support literature currently available; and finally, in the memorial strategies of queer parents in our studies.

QUEER EXPERIENCES OF REPRODUCTIVE LOSS

Although there are many similarities in the experiences of all grieving parents, queer experiences of loss are often intensified by homophobic and heteronormative treatment by healthcare practitioners as well as family and coworkers. Sometimes this occurs outright—several participants in our survey and interviews shared stories of partners being forced to wait outside while they were given the news of a loss, and one had to make burial arrangements alone for a stillborn child. Yet even for those who did not feel they experienced homophobia during their loss, their fear of homophobia frequently kept them from accessing resources such as local loss support groups, which other researchers have shown to be helpful to many heterosexual couples (see Linda Layne's *Motherhood Lost*).

Although the adoption industry offers few statistics on "failed adoptions," experiences of having children "reclaimed" by birth-parents following adoption placement are devastating. Indeed, these interviews suggest that these difficult experiences may be more likely for LGBTQ families because of homophobia and heterosexism within adoption agencies and among birth families. For instance, several parents explained that the birthmother's decision to "reclaim" the child was influenced by her family's discomfort. As one gay male adoptive parent mimicked tearfully, "I don't want faggots raising my grandchild." This complicates the popular "reassurance" narratives adoption agencies often put forth to prospective queer clients, of bioparents who want their children to have the presumed affluence associated (particularly) with gay male adoptive parents.

In the academic literature, studies of queer reproduction and parenting have also been prevalent in the past few decades, yet most make only brief mention of miscarriages and failed adoptions. We review these in greater detail in "Stories of Grief and Hope: Queer Experiences of Reproductive Loss" (Craven and Peel), but for the purposes of this chapter, we will only detail those address-ing reproductive loss as their primary focus. The first empirical study of lesbian experiences of pregnancy loss was published in 2007 by Danuta Wojnar, a nurse, in a midwifery journal. This small qualitative study drew on interviews with ten white lesbian couples in the USA, all of whom had planned their pregnancies. (She notes that about 50 percent of heterosexuals' pregnancies are unplanned; 483). Wojnar found that, unlike some heterosexual mothers, lesbian mothers frequently bonded with their unborn child early in pregnancy (Wojnar 482).

Michelle Walks has addressed the topic of infertility in queer families, noting in particular the flawed logic of previous studies that highlighted the "fairly unique advantage" for lesbian women, in that if one partner was unable to conceive (or experienced a miscarriage), they could "swap" (Dunne 26). Walks emphasizes the emotional challenges that such an arrangement posed for some queer couples, especially "people who do not embrace a stereo-typical 'feminine' identity, such as butches, genderqueers, or some trans-identified individuals" (Walks 138).

Joanne Cacciatore and Zulma Raffo published a study on "same-gender (homosexual) bereaved parents" in the journal *Social Work* in 2011. Through interviews with six white lesbian parents, they explore the intersection of what they term "stigmatized re-lationships" and "stigmatized deaths." Bereaved lesbian mothers experience a double disenfranchisement, since not only do they experience a dearth of support for their experiences with loss, but they may also avoid support services that require them to explain or justify their family. For all six participants, the authors note that "ritual and remembrance—including things from hand molds to memorial services—appeared to play a key role in the integration of loss [into their lives as the 'new normal']" (Cacciatore and Raffo 174), which is a point we will return to below.

The publication of data from Elizabeth's online survey in 2010 was the first major empirical study addressing queer women's ex-periences of pregnancy loss. Among other findings, 85 percent of mothers (both social and biological) felt that their loss—whether it occurred early or late in the pregnancy—had a "significant" or "very significant" impact on their lives. Furthermore, the experi-ence of loss for lesbian and bisexual women was amplified because of the emotional and financial investment respondents reported making in their impending motherhood, and the heterosexism some experienced from health professionals.

The publication of self-help books for parents and professionals on achieving conception, pursuing adoption and surrogacy, and parenting in queer families has also boomed in the past decade. This LGBTQ parenting literature—primarily in the form of guides for conception, pregnancy, surrogacy, and adoption—are notably neglectful in discussing loss, frequently devoting only a sidebar or a few pages to the possibility, if they discuss it at all. For instance, of the top 10 hits in a search of www.amazon.com for LGBTQ conception, pregnancy, adoption, and surrogacy guides, only two discussed miscarriage explicitly (Martin 258; Pepper).[2] This not only speaks to a broader societal discomfort with the notion of loss, but also contributes to a narrative of achieving queer families in a cultural and political moment that frequently hypervalues nuclear, heterosexual family formation. As Petra Nordqvist and Carol Smart argue (albeit in a primarily heterosexual context), "British society (along with many others in the West) has undergone a kind of 'geneticisation' of the popular imagination, such that now genes are increasingly believed to be of overwhelming significance in every aspect of life" (4). This is abundantly clear in the dearth of support resources available for LGBTQ bereaved parents, especially non-gestational parents.

Most self-help material on reproductive loss is geared toward heterosexual, married (often white, middle class, and Christian) couples—in fact, none of the top ten hits in a search for "miscarriage" mention LGBTQ experiences at all, nor do those for adoption. The scarcity of support materials on lesbian and bisexual women's experiences with reproductive loss is only magnified in the dearth of materials on reproductive loss for gay and bisexual men pursuing adoption or surrogacy (Riggs et al.), or the reproductive losses of transgender and other queer parents (Walks). The minimal resources available offer little support for grieving reproductive losses, nor memorializing these experiences in ways that acknowledge and support queer identities and communities.

MEMORIALIZATION OF REPRODUCTIVE LOSS IN LGBTQ COMMUNITIES: A BEGINNING

Little has been written on memorialization of LGBTQ experiences with reproductive loss. Cacciatore and Raffo present four brief quotes describing lesbian parents' experiences participating in rituals—such as making a birthday cake for their child each year, wearing a locket with their child's photo, sculpting their child's face in clay, and getting commemorative memorial tattoos.

In Elizabeth's survey, questions asked whether the respondents kept mementos or "keepsakes"—such as ultrasound scans, locks of hair, ID bracelets, foot or hand prints, or birth and/or death certificates—and whether they had a memorial of any kind, such as a service, funeral, planted a tree, or do anything to acknowledge the birth date. Nine respondents (15 percent of the survey sample) indicated that they had kept an ultrasound scan of their child; eight

(13 percent) kept their child's clothes, a lock of hair, hand or foot prints, and ID bracelet or photos following stillbirths; and six (10 percent) retained a birth and/or death certificate. One respondent expressed regret that she had not kept a scan of her child: "We were offered a scan picture at the time and refused—with hindsight I probably would have liked to have it." Following the loss, nine respondents (15 percent) kept their mementos privately in a box or drawer, and several noted returning to them to read or feel them. Five (8 percent) displayed photos and other mementos publically in their home. None threw them away.

Ten respondents (17 percent) reported having a memorial service—some private, others with family and/or community. Several buried or spread the ashes of their child, one Jewish couple said kaddish, and several planted trees or bushes in the child's honour, which they continue to visit. Although not asked explicitly, several noted remembering the children in some way on their birthday each year. One respondent who had experienced two losses remarked, "I often feel there should be marks on my body to reflect these pregnancies having happened, and am considering a pair of tattoos/scars/piercings," but had concern about turning her body into "a tally of loss."

In Christa's interviews, nearly half of the participants (n=21) had a physical memorial of some kind; nearly one-third (n=14) had a ceremony dedicated to their child; and 20 percent (n=10) had a commemorative tattoo to mark their experience and/or memorialize their child's life. What is important regarding the study of LGBTQ experiences with reproductive loss, and the memorialization of reproductive loss more broadly, is that many of these memorials—particularly those that engaged the parents' communities or were displayed publically—allowed parents to mourn their loss or losses with and within their communities. One participant, Anna,[3] described what she felt was an enhanced need to memorialize reproductive loss experiences within queer communities.

> Anna: In the queer community, there is more need for ceremony around the loss than in the straight community.
> Christa: Why do you think that?

Anna: Because there is so much of our experiences that get invisiblized. And I think that there are ways in which the queer community has had to find ways to make our experiences valid or to ritualize things or to make them just as important as straight experiences.

For Anna, a white pagan lesbian, and her Jewish partner Jude, that ritual took the form of a ceremony made by a friend, an interfaith minister. The ceremony that the minister (and close friend) designed for Anna and Jude, and their son Kaleb, who was three at the time, honoured their loss of Josie, their adopted daughter who had been part of their family for five days before her birthmother reclaimed her. Prior to their loss, their minister had begun to knit a hat for Josie, but it remained unfinished when she left Anna, Jude, and Kaleb's family. Initially, their minister proposed finishing the hat and giving it to Anna and Jude as a gift for a future child. Unsure at

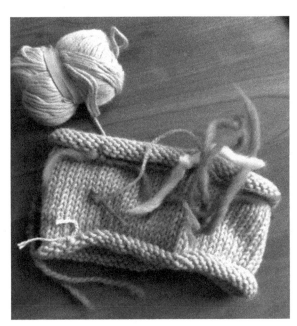

the time whether they would enter into the adoption process again— although they did later adopt a second son—Anna asked that the hat remain Josie's. As a tribute to the strong, primarily lesbian, community that supported their family through the loss, those who attended the ceremony were each asked to add a piece of string

Figure 1

to contribute to the memorial. During our interview at her home, Anna walked to a nearby desk and brought out this hat, and noted that even seven years after the loss, she kept Josie's hat close to her every day (Figure 1).[4]

Nora and Alex's memorial was also a powerful one (Figure 2). After Nora, a cisgender lesbian, physically experienced a loss and later developed health complications that made another pregnancy dangerous for her, Nora and Alex decided that Alex, who previously identified as FTM and now genderqueer, would carry their next child. The experience of becoming a "social mother" after carrying their first child was also complicated for Nora, as she explained in the interview.

> In losing our daughter and in making the decision that it wouldn't be safe for me to carry again, and because we live in [a US state that prohibits listing two same-sex parents on a birth certificate], I lost not only a biological and a physical connection and the possibility of breastfeeding my, our first child ... I also lost the ability to have legal

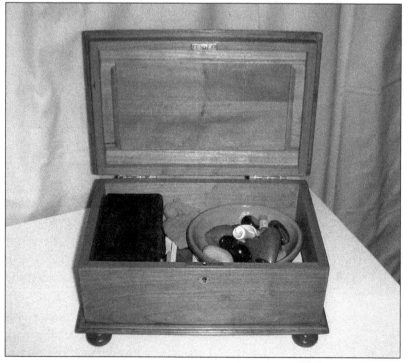

Figure 2

[rights to our future children], to have my name on this child's birth certificate ... I'm not even going to be able to petition for that [where we live].

Nora's losses were multiplied by the homophobic laws that will now govern her relationship—or lack of legal relationship—with her child born by her partner. The memorials they created also speak to the depth of their experience of losing their daughter Hayden at eight weeks. This memory box holds a remembrance bowl for Hayden. It sits prominently in their bedroom beside the urn that holds her ashes, along with the sentiments that friends and family wrote during a ceremony to honour Hayden.

Many participants also shared the birth announcements that they had made for the child or children that they had lost, as well as their subsequent children, which served as a commemoration for themselves and their community. Giovanna, a single lesbian mother from Italy, sent the following birth announcement to her friends and family, following the death and birth of her eight-month-old son, Jacob.

In loving memory of my beautiful and perfect baby boy
Conceived on May 8th, 2010
Flew away with the angels on January 10th, 2011
Was born sleeping on January 11th, 2011
Was due on February 7th, 2011
...
I will forever be proud of my beloved son,
Your existence inside me gave me the happiest and
most wonderful 8 months of my life. I am grateful
we shared so much during the short time we had together.
My life will never be the same again.

Thank you [Jacob], I will miss you so much,
ti amo pulciacchiotto,
La tua mamma

Thalia, a lesbian mother from Canada, sent the following birth announcement with the words to "You are my Sunshine" printed on the reverse.

> To deny our grief is to deny our love—for we loved her way before she was here
>
> ...
>
> Thank you for sharing in our joy when we were expecting [Rachel]
> And for sharing in the sorrow of losing our little girl.
> We hurt knowing that she never got to see how many people
> were looking forward to meeting and loving her.

Others posted their memories and requests to social media, a medium that scholars have described as a form of "self-documentation," an "extension" of forms such as personal diaries, snapshots, and even formal autobiographies (Kitzman 44). Online forums also frequently serve as a space for what sociologists Deborah Davidson and Gayle Letherby describe as "griefwork" among bereaved parents and their support communities (214). For instance, Karrie—a lesbian mother of four, who lives with her partner Stacia in a rural US community with few other LGBTQ families in her immediate circle of friends—posted the following on Facebook:

KARRIE SANDS

It's October 16th again. Eight years ago today, I held my beautiful baby girl in my arms, and tried to figure out how to say hello and goodbye all at once.

This morning I sat down with [my twins], and told them the story of their oldest sister. (It's something I did with [Arielle, my second daughter] when she was an infant, too.) I know it will be years before they understand, but for now, I want them to have heard. I want them to know that this family is bigger than just what they see. I want them to know who she is, and why she's important. I want her to know, too—she must know, wherever she is—how much she is remembered and loved...

As we do each fall, we will make a birthday donation in her name. This year, the charity we have chosen is MyStuff. Children who are taken from abusive situations to shelters or foster care often must leave behind all their belongings. MyStuff provides kids in crisis with a duffel bag full of toys, books, toiletries, a stuffed animal and a blanket. Their goal is to provide a bag to each of the 300,000 children who face these situations each year. You can join us in celebrating [Sammy's] life with your own donation, at www.mystuffbags.org.

It's hard to believe eight whole years have gone by. When I close my eyes, it feels like just yesterday. Nothing—nothing—will ever erase the love I feel for this precious child. Having the chance, however brief, to be her mother, far outweighs the pain of losing her.

Happy Birthday, precious child. You will live on forever in my heart.

Karrie and Stacia lost Samantha at term (just before forty weeks), and each year, they pick a different charity to support—and encourage their friends and family to do so—in her memory. The post above received many "likes" and sentiments of support from friends and family, which attests to the forms of community that can support families experiencing loss.

To mark what would have been the second birthday of her son, Giovanna, who was introduced above, sent the following e-card to friends and family that read:

Today ... is my son's [Jacob's] second birthday: I would like to remember and commemorate him with joy and gratefulness and not just with sadness and longing, would you want to help me? In this case, could you do a "random act of kindness" in [Jacob's] name and let me know about it? These will be his birthday presents from all of you! This good deed could be towards a human being, an animal, a donation to an association ... anything that comes to your mind!

Giovanna also included her first son in the birth announcement she mailed to family and friends for her subsequent son Joshua, keeping the memory of the child she lost integral to the vision of family she sought to convey to her community of family and friends: "[Joshua's] big brother and guardian angel [Jacob] will always be with us." Both of these examples express a public (re)acknowledgement of loss that was important in many of the interviews, and indicates an engagement with community around grief and queer experience. Others created physical memorials themselves to honour their children. Amelia and Selena, queer and bisexual women (respectively) living in an urban neighborhood, developed a free lending library that they placed in front of their home in honour of their living son, and their son who was stillborn at thirty-eight weeks (Figure 3).

Figure 3

Michelle and Char—lesbian women who had divorced after experiencing a twelve-week loss but remain committed to co-parenting their subsequent twins—made a more private memorial with an icicle ornament that they hung together each year at the top of their Christmas tree in honour of their first child (Figure 4).

Although ceremonies and physical memorials appeared more common for children who had passed away later during a preg-

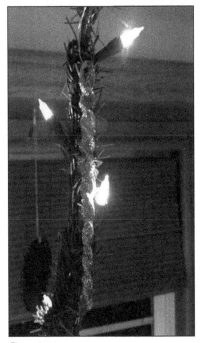

Figure 4

nancy, or who were removed following an adoption placement, parents with a wide variety of reproductive experiences chose to memorialize their experience with tattoos. For instance, Nora and Alex, introduced above, envisioned matching tattoos to mark their experience together. Nora's iris, inked on almost the full length of her back, was a significant commitment of remembrance for their daughter. Alex explained: "we both would ultimately like to get the iris tattoo. Nora got it right before I got pregnant, and so I plan on getting it after I finish breastfeeding" (Figure 5).

Leah and Jessica, from Maryland, got matching tattoos of the Hebrew transliteration of the letters "V-V-L-B-Y" for Wallaby, which is what they called their unborn baby. Jessica wrote about this experience in an email. "A friend of ours, upon seeing it (because handwritten Hebrew can be so subjective), said: 'Before reading that it was 'Vallabee,' I read it as: 'oo-levei,' or, 'of my heart.' That always made me happy too." In this case, their tattoos have functioned not only as a memorial but as part of their long-term healing and their connection to wider communities of support (Figure 6).

As Deborah Davidson writes in the introduction to *The Tattoo Project*—a 2016 edited collection featuring analysis of "The Tattoo Project," the online digital archive of commemorative tattoos, by archivists, social scientists, and digital humanists—"tattoos puncture and disrupt; what was once unseen appears" (1). Tattoos

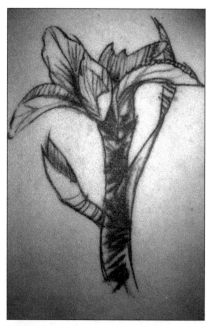

Figure 5

commemorating reproductive loss offer possibilities for managing grief and engagement with community, particularly when they do not outwardly resemble a memorial as other commemorative tattoos that include more identifiable details (such as birth and death dates for a loved one) can. Many memorial tattoos representing experiences of reproductive loss are symbolic and hold a subjective meaning to their bearer—a way for "the griever to seek and receive support from others" (Davidson and Duhig 66).

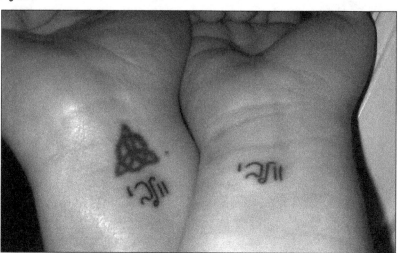

Figure 6

In this context, it is significant to note that almost all of the memorial tattoos are in public, visible places on participants' bodies—even if not always identifiable to someone who does not know their experience. This suggests that the grieving process is a communal one, especially in the ways bereaved parents have shared the meanings of their tattoos with others. As Andreas Kitzman writes of commemorative tattoos about loss or trauma: "[they can function] as conduits for autobiographical narratives to pass through. They remain closed when necessary, but once opened by permission of the host, allow for meaningful exchange of cherished memories and the recantations of life-changing events" (43).

As with those Davidson interviewed in her research on grief and bereavement, it was common among those Christa interviewed to emphasize the importance of talking about death and the child they lost, despite—and sometimes because of—the social taboo of talking about death and adoptive loss. This was particularly heightened for LGBTQ parents who shared concerns about not only the taboo of talking about death and grief but also their efforts to create families outside of heteronormative expectations. Deborah Davidson and Angelina Duhig write:

> Talking about one's tattoo becomes a method to maintain a memory of someone in our external environment but also introduce this person to new acquaintances by bringing knowledge of their existence into our new relationships. The tattoo allows the bearer to do this with more ease, as the image can normalize conversations about something that would otherwise be a difficult dialogue, and serves as an intuitively yet universally experienced channel whereby this becomes possible. (89)

Although many LGBTQ participants did find ways to normalize conversations about their experiences of reproductive loss, some were also cautious about doing so in spaces where they were concerned about a homophobic response. Most had alternative or generalized explanations of their tattoos ready to share as well.

Some commemorative tattoos also incorporated all of the participant's children. Danielle, a femme lesbian, has this tattoo on her foot with the Latin words for "Let your light shine" (Figure 7). The sun and the moon represent her twins, five years old at the time of the interview, and the three stars represent three of her losses. She had plans to add a fourth star for her most recent miscarriage.

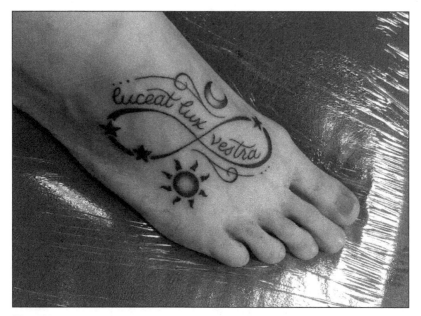

Figure 7

The continued griefwork that the permanency of memorial tattoos encourages creates a form of embodied memorialization extending far beyond the individual or family that has experienced the loss. In fact, contributors to *The Tattoo Project* found that commemorative tattoos—including memorials but also other life events, such as survival after sexual assault, educational achievements, spiritual connections, military service, self-forgiveness, and friendship—are relatively common. Tattoo artists interviewed for the book estimated commemorative tattoos represented from 50 percent to 90 percent of all tattoos (6-7).

A significant aspect of commemorative tattoos, which cannot be explored fully here, is that they were accessible to parents across the socioeconomic spectrum. Although a memorial tattoo often costs several hundred dollars, a full burial service frequently costs several thousand. Anthropologist Ken Colson has suggested that the association of tattoos with "low status and marginal or deviant occupations and behaviors" (18) has limited research on memorial tattooing. Yet his research on tattoo testimonials from major tattoo magazines in the United States uncovered what he termed "conventional motifs" (such as the icons and epitaphs common on

240

gravestones) and "unconventional motifs," often stylized tattoos that were indistinguishable from other tattoos unless the bearer shared their meaning (Colson 18). For many participants in our research, tattoos with "unconventional motifs" offered a relatively low-cost, but high-impact commitment to memorializing their experience and to managing support from others, as they chose to share or not share the meaning behind it.

In a final example, Tanea also incorporated her experience of loss into an existing tattoo incorporating part of a quote from Langston Hughes, "Free within Ourselves" and birds in flight encircling her forearm, that had important meaning for her as a Black, queer woman (Figures 8 and 9). She explained this in the interview:

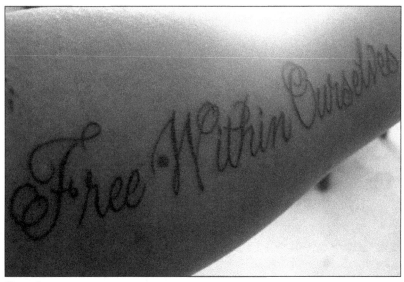

Figure 8

> When people ask about the meaning, it's sometimes easier just to focus on the words, as they apply to race and sexuality and the freedom to be true to oneself, loving yourself in spite of the obstacles before you. The birds are meant to connect to those words and ideas, but for me th[ey] have another meaning, too. During my pregnancy, images of birds kept coming up for me, and I felt that they represented, in a way, the next chapter of my life. I was planning on

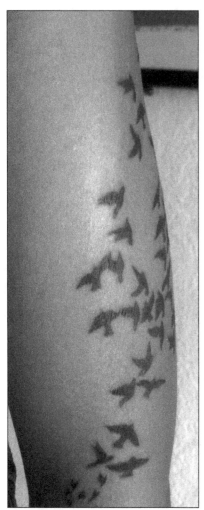

Figure 9

decorating the baby's room with birds, and for a while, I was considering getting a dove tattoo after the baby was born. Of course, all of that symbolism shifted when the baby died. But these birds still represent to me new life, unconditional love for self and others, and freedom. They remind me that I don't have to let go of all of the positive changes the baby brought to my life— changes like focusing more on self-care than I ever had before, and trusting in the path I'm walking, even if I meet unexpected turns. And the act itself, of putting this art permanently on my body, also holds meaning, as this baby's love was so special to me, and I know it will never leave me.

For Tanea, part of her healing process toward "freedom" and "loving [her]self" was letting go of an abusive relationship with an ex-boyfriend she had been in when the baby was conceived. As she explains, her tattoo holds multiple meanings, and like many of the others presented above, ones that she can choose whether to share with others.

CONCLUSION

Creative responses to loss represent a beginning for many LGBTQ families, not merely the end of a life they cherished. The beginning often takes the form of seeking support and conversation within their communities. Rodríguez's call to reconfigure an understanding of queer sexual politics with consideration of both utopian longings and everyday failures resonates with memorializing queer reproductive loss in important ways. Creativity in memorialization offers one space within with to challenge heteronormative, and even homonormative, notions of family formation. Reproductive futures for queer families that incorporate grief, sorrow, longing, and loss have the potential to destabilize "success" narratives in a political moment that valorizes nuclear families within queer communities. The examples in our research suggest that the possibilities for memorialization of reproductive loss can push the boundaries of identity, notions of family, and experiences of grief that serve an important role in queer reproductive experience.

ENDNOTES

[1]The terminology here—as with much discussion of queer identity and experiences of reproductive loss—is imperfect. Some researchers prefer "social" mother/parent or "other mother" to identify a parent who did not experience a physical pregnancy, although we feel that these identifiers downplay the shared parenting role. Additionally, in the age of assisted reproduction, a "social" parent may indeed be biologically related to a child if in-vitro fertilization was used or a family member donated sperm. Similarly using "non-biological" can also be inaccurate. We settle on "non-gestational" in this chapter to highlight the ways in which being pregnant, particularly the physical appearance of pregnancy and its subsequent absence in the case of second and third trimester pregnancy loss, infuses the experiences of some queer parents differently than others.

[2]Many thanks to Christa's research assistants Edie Anderson, Jacob Danko, and Abigail Boll for contributing to the search for this information.

[3]All names, including those of family members, are pseudonyms. Demographic data is provided for context and where relevant to the participant's experience, but it is limited in order to preserve confidentiality.

[4]Many interview participants generously donated photographs

and announcements to include in this project. Christa Craven collected each image and received written permission for its use in publications from the creator. In the interests of maintaining confidentiality, no formal attribution is provided.

WORKS CITED

Cacciatore, Joanne, and Zulma Raffo. "An Exploration of Lesbian Maternal Bereavement." *Social Work*, vol. 56, no. 2, 2011, pp. 169-177.

Colson, Ken. "Tattooing and Death: An American Folk Custom." *Teaching Anthropology: Society for Anthropology in Community Colleges Notes*, vol. 4, no. 2, 1997, pp. 18-23.

Craven, Christa, and Elizabeth Peel. "Stories of Grief and Hope: Queer Experiences of Reproductive Loss." *Queering Motherhood: Narrative and Theoretical Perspectives*, edited by Margaret Gibson, Demeter Press, 2014, pp. 97-110.

Davidson, Deborah, and Angelina Duhig. "Visual Research Methods: Memorial Tattoos as Memory-Realization." *The Tattoo Project: Commemorative Tattoos, Visual Culture, and the Digital Archive*, edited by Deborah Davidson, Canadian Scholars' Press, 2016, pp. 63–75.

Davidson, Deborah, and Gayle Letherby. "Griefwork Online: Perinatal Loss, Lifecourse Disruption and Online Support." *Human Fertility*, vol. 17, no. 3, 2014, pp. 214-217.

Davidson, Deborah, editor. *The Tattoo Project: Commemorative Tattoos, Visual Culture and the Digital Archive*. Canadian Scholars' Press, 2017.

Davidson, Deborah. "The Tattoo Project at York University." *The Tattoo Project,* thetattooproject.info. Accessed 14 Sept. 2017.

Dunne, Gillian A. "Opting into Motherhood: Lesbians Blurring the Boundaries and Transforming the Meaning of Parenthood and Kinship." *Gender and Society*, vol. 14, no. 1, 2000, pp. 11-35.

Halberstam, J. *The Queer Art of Failure*. Duke University Press, 2011.

Kitzmann, Andreas. "Between the Inside and the Outside: Commemorative Tattoos and the Externalization of Loss and Trauma." *The Tattoo Project: Commemorative Tattoos, Visual Culture, and the Digital Archive*, edited by Deborah Davidson, Canadian Scholars' Press, 2016, pp. 39–47.

Layne, Linda L. *Motherhood Lost: A Feminist Account of Pregnancy Loss in America*. Routledge, 2003.

Love, Heather. *Feeling Backward: Loss and the Politics of Queer History*. Harvard University Press, 2009.

Martin, April. *The Lesbian and Gay Parenting Handbook: Creating and Raising Our Families*. HarperPerennial, 1993.

Nordqvist, Petra, and Carol Smart. *Relative Strangers: Family Life, Genes and Donor Conception*. Palgrave Macmillan, 2014.

Peel, Elizabeth. "Pregnancy Loss in Lesbian and Bisexual Women: An Online Survey of Experiences." *Human Reproduction*, vol. 25, no. 3, 2010, pp. 721-27.

Peel, Elizabeth, and Ruth Cain. "Silent Miscarriage and Deafening Heteronormativity: An Experiential and Critical Feminist Account." *Understanding Reproductive Loss: International Perspectives on Life, Death and Fertility*, edited by S. Earle et al., Ashgate, 2012, pp. 79-92.

Pepper, Rachel. *The Ultimate Guide to Pregnancy for Lesbians: How to Stay Sane and Care for Yourself from Pre-Conception through Birth*, 2nd ed. Cleis Press, 2005.

Riggs, Damien W. et al. "Gay Men's Experiences of Surrogacy Clinics in India." *Journal of Family Planning and Reproductive Health Care*, vol. 41, no. 1, 2015, pp. 48–53.

Rodríguez, Juana María. *Sexual Futures, Queer Gestures, and Other Latina Longings*. New York University Press, 2014.

Walks, Michelle. "Breaking the Silence: Infertility, Motherhood, and Queer Culture." *Journal of the Association for Research on Mothering. Special Issue: Mothering, Race, Ethnicity, Culture, and Class*, vol. 9, no. 2, 2007, pp. 130-143.

Wojnar, Danuta. "Miscarriage Experiences of Lesbian Couples." *Journal of Midwifery & Women's Health*, vol. 52, no. 5, 2007, pp. 479-85.

About the Contributors

Maya Bhave's PhD (Loyola University, Chicago) focused on Ethiopian immigrant women, capital, and the informal economy. She taught sociology at North Park University for ten years before moving to Vermont. Her current research interests are the following: life, work, and family balance; gender identity among female soccer players and female coaches; adoption and feminist identity; and motherhood and child loss. She teaches as an adjunct professor at St. Michael's College and lives with her husband and two sons near Burlington, Vermont.

Miriam Rose Brooker was awarded her PhD in 2016. Her thesis entitled, Lilith's daughters: Women's experiences of healing after abortion was awarded the Edith Cowan University Magdalena Prize for Feminist Research. Miriam's thesis drew on feminist body scholarship, phenomenology, and art-based research practices to generate an innovative methodology designed to sensitively elicit embodied stories of the abortion experience and its aftermath, and the visual, symbolic and non-verbal expressions that accompanied them.

Christa Craven is an Associate Professor of Anthropology and Women's, Gender, and Sexuality Studies at the College of Wooster in Ohio, USA. She is the author of Pushing for Midwives: Homebirth Mothers and the Reproductive Rights Movement (2010), co-author of *Feminist Ethnography: Thinking Through Methodologies, Challenges & Possibilities* (with Dána-Ain Davis,

2016), and co-editor of the collection *Feminist Activist Ethnography: Counterpoints to Neoliberalism in North America* (also with Davis, 2013). Craven is former co-chair of the Society of Lesbian and Gay Anthropologists (now the Association for Queer Anthropology).

Angie Deveau is a graduate of York University's Women's Studies MA Program and currently works for the Motherhood Initiative for Research and Community Involvement and Demeter Press. Previously, she provided research assistance for York University's Gender and Work Database; York University's "Women's Human Rights, Macroeconomics and Policy Choices" project; and the "Adolescent Health and Wellbeing Study" at the University of New Brunswick. In addition to her background in research, Angie has worked as a case management assistant for the Province of Nova Scotia's Department of Community Services, and as the community development coordinator for the Victorian Order of Nurses/Help the Aged project in Fredericton, New Brunswick.

Nancy Gerber received her doctorate in English from Rutgers University and taught for eight years in the English and Women's Studies Departments at Rutgers University-Newark. She is currently enrolled in a psychoanalytic training program at the Academy of Clinical and Applied Psychoanalysis. Her work has appeared in feminist anthologies, including *Moms Gone Mad: Motherhood and Madness, Oppression and Resistance* (Demeter 2012), and *The M Word: Real Mothers in Contemporary Art* (Demeter 2011). Her most recent book is *Fire and Ice: Poetry and Prose* (Arseya 2014).

Keren Epstein-Gilboa is a registered nurse and registered psychotherapist with a PhD in developmental psychology. She is a Lamaze certified childbirth educator and a board certified lactation consultant. Her clinical work includes individual, couple, and family psychotherapy as well as childbirth and lactation support. She is also a university lecturer and teaches courses in psychology. She has several publications related to the psychology of the female physiological continuum and maternal, paternal, infant, child, and family development.

Elizabeth Heineman has been at the University of Iowa since 1999 and teaches courses on Germany, Europe, gender, and human rights. Her research has examined gender, war, and memory; welfare states in comparative perspective; the significance of marital status for women; the erotica industry; gender and human rights; and pregnancy and infant loss; and the politics of maternal health care. She currently serves as the chair of the Department of History.

Brittany Irvine is a perinatal-paediatric epidemiologist and doula working in the Ottawa area. She holds a Masters of Arts in Religious Studies where her scholarly focus was on feminist studies and relations of power, cultural accommodation in childbirth, birthing rituals and shamanic traditions. After completing a Graduate Certificate in Population Health Risk Assessment and Management from the University of Ottawa, her work became mostly quantitative, focused on rare perinatal and neonatal-paediatric disease surveillance. Her hope is to develop a research portfolio which may bridge the gap between feminist cultural studies about midwifery and epidemiology.

Rhobi Jacobs is a Canadian-born social worker and birth care provider practising and residing in the Greater Toronto Area. Her autobiographical works of creative nonfiction and poetry feature the nuances of life in subrural Ontario. She is the mother of three live children and one babe she looks forward to meeting in the Hereafter.

Emily R.M. Lind is a doctoral candidate at Carleton University's Institute for Comparative Studies in Literature, Art, and Culture. Her research examines the intersections between identity, materiality, power, and knowledge production in interdisciplinary contexts. She is currently writing her dissertation on settler colonialism, Canadian art, and early twentieth-century Toronto.

Natalie Morning is a Learning Strategist and part-time instructor at Ryerson University. She is a graduate of the joint Communication and Culture Master's program at York University and Ryerson

University. Her research interests concern motherless daughters and art as a tool for community building, parental loss, memoir writing, post-secondary pathways for non-traditional students, motherhood ambivalence, and feminist considerations of mothering.

Maria Novotny is a PhD student in rhetoric and writing at Michigan State University. Her area of study is in cultural rhetorics, focusing on rhetorics of motherhood, pregnancy, and infertility. She further studies public rhetoric, focusing on the legislation advocating for reproductive and adoption rights.

Rachel O'Donnell is a mother who experienced baby loss and a PhD Candidate in political science at York University, Toronto. She is a fiction writer and is working on a dissertation on the feminist politics of botanical exploration and women's knowledge of fertility plant properties in Latin America. She is originally from Pennsylvania and is a U.S. citizen and Canadian resident.

Elizabeth Peel is a Professor of Communication and Social Interaction at Loughborough University, UK. Her most recent books are *Ageing & Sexualities* (with Rosie Harding) and *Critical Kinship Studies* (with Damien W. Riggs). She is a Fellow of the British Psychological Society and edits, with Elizabeth Stokoe, the Routledge 'Gender and Sexualities in Psychology' book series.

Margie Serrato is a cultural anthropologist. Her doctoral thesis focused on issues of gender and sexuality in the post-9/11 U.S. military context, but her research extends more generally to gender in cross-cultural perspectives, organizational contexts, and educational settings. Margie's recent work includes efforts to broaden underrepresented participation in STEM fields.

Robin Silbergleid is the author of *The Baby Book* and the memoir *Texas Girl* (Demeter 2014). In addition to publishing on reproductive loss, she regularly participates with the international art, oral history, and portraiture project The ART of Infertility. She is associate professor of English at Michigan State University.

j wallace skelton thinks the compulsory gender binary harms all of us, and is interj wallace skelton thinks the compulsory gender binary harms all of us, and is interested in creating more possibilities and autonomy for everyone. j works for the Toronto District School Board's Gender Based Violence Prevention Office and is a PhD student at OISE, co-researching with children how they imagine school that would celebrate gender diversity. j's recent publications include *Transphobia, Deal With It and be a Gender Transcender* and *The Last Place You Look* for children, and academic writing in *Trans Studies Quarterly, Education Canada* and an assortment of anthologies. j identifies as queer and trans, parents three children, and is well loved.

Mindy Stricke is an award-winning photographer and interdisciplinary community artist whose collaborative practice blends photography, documentary audio, writing, collage, sculpture, and performance. Her most recent project, *Grief Landscapes,* a photographic exploration of people's experiences with grief and bereavement, was awarded a 2016 Visual Arts Grant from the Ontario Arts Council. Her previous series of participatory art projects, *Greetings From Motherland,* brought mothers together to make work that challenged traditional representations of motherhood, and was awarded grants from the Toronto Arts Council, the Ontario Arts Council and the Canada Council for the Arts. *The Greetings From Motherland* project "Good Eater" was featured in *At The Table: Mothers Sharing Their Stories Through Art,* a documentary short by filmmaker Brijetta Hall Waller. Mindy's photographs and installations have been exhibited throughout North America, and featured in *The New York Times, Time, Newsweek, Japan's Voce, Toronto Star, Modern Loss, What's Your Grief,* and the Smithsonian Institute Photography Initiative's book and online exhibit, *Click! Photography Changes Everything.* Originally from New York, she now lives in Toronto with her husband and two children.

Masha Sukovic, PhD, is a writer and a professor at the University of Utah. Her areas of expertise include women's and gender studies, performance studies, health communication, qualitative methods, intercultural communication, and creative writing. Her current research interests involve arts-based research; study of race, ethnicity, and immigrant identities; narrative inquiry in health contexts; and issues pertaining to motherhood, gender, sexuality, culture, and food.

Mary Thompson is associate professor of English at James Madison University where she also coordinates the Women's and Gender Studies Program. She teaches courses in women's literature, feminist theory, and women's and Gender Studies. Her research examines popular and literary representations of reproductive justice issues.